Laugh With Kathy

Finding Humor in the Journey through Breast Cancer

KATHY LARIVIERE

DEDICATION

To Dad—who always wanted me to write a book.

To the loves of my life—Gene, Nicholas, Steven, Danielle, and Samantha.

To my mother—whom I could talk to about anything.

To my friend Tess—who always picked up the phone and made me laugh, got into trouble with me, and kept me out of jail.

To Chris, Julie, and Brad—the best cancer mentors.

To my health-care providers—who walked this journey with me.

To my many friends and family who drove me to my appointments, watched me sleep, and laughed with me along the way.

And to the one in eight women who will experience breast cancer in their lifetimes.

CONTENTS

PREFACE

There is nothing funny about being diagnosed with cancer. Thanks to improvements in treatments and research, more and more people are surviving cancer. But for me, simply surviving was not enough. I didn't want to just survive cancer; I wanted to crush it. Since I couldn't do that, the next best thing was to laugh at it. After all, what could be more demoralizing to an enemy than to laugh at them? This book is intended to be a lighthearted, quirky look at surviving breast cancer.

I originally wrote Laugh with Kathy as a blog while I was going through the diagnosis and treatment of breast cancer. I used the blog to sort out and share my experiences with my friends and family. Over time, more and more people started following the blog and asking me to convert it into book format so that they could share it with others. But it wasn't until I started getting e-mails from other breast cancer patients telling me I had made their day that I considered publishing a book.

Most of the writing in this book comes directly from the blog, with only minor clarifications or grammatical corrections. I have added some new posts that were never published on the blog. Some of the new posts are retrospective in nature, while others I wrote during treatment and never published because I wasn't ready to share them at the time.

The original blog posts were written in chronological order as the events occurred. But for the book, I chose to rearrange the posts into chapters by subject so that I could focus on one topic at a time. Most entries are in chronological order, except for those that needed to be moved for clarification. Since some of my treatments overlapped (radiation therapy and chemo phase three in particular) or were over extended periods of time, I have included dates as a reference.

CHAPTER 1
DISCOVERY AND DIAGNOSIS

As a teenager, I dreamed of writing like Erma Bombeck. Her ability to write about everyday life and make us laugh inspired me to write. She, too, was diagnosed with breast cancer, but did not live long enough to share that journey with us. I would like to think she would have faced it much the same way as I have, by writing about that journey and laughing along the way.

My journey with breast cancer started on a beautiful fall day in Iowa. Little did I know that my life was about to be turned upside down. Life was good. I was fifty-two years old and married to the man who had been my friend, lover, and companion for twenty-nine years. My three children were grown and "off the family payroll," and my thirteen-year-old sheltie, Dolly Dog, walked beside me on the driveway as we looked over the Cedar River and viewed the changing fall colors. I simply could not imagine the difficult journey I was about to undertake. Nor could I imagine how much humor I would find in the diagnosis, treatment, and survival of the disease.

If you ask them, my friends and family will tell you that I have always been creative in how I celebrate life. When my children were young, I would invent crazy math and science projects for them to learn from over summer break. Now that they are grown, every Christmas I plan a fun competition for them, including cooking challenges, birdhouse building, Lego scene constructing, or quizzes on family history, all with fun prizes for the winners. My friends are sometimes confused by my creative party invitations, including one invitation in the form of a subpoena, which caused one friend to contact her attorney.

Sometimes that creativity has gotten me into trouble, like the time I poked fun at Homeland Security on my blog, and they e-mailed me about my comments. My best friend, Tess, is an attorney, and I called her in a panic when I received the e-mail. When she finally quit laughing, she advised me to stay off the Internet for a couple of weeks and not reply to the e-mail. I tried, I really did, but the Homeland Security contact finally called me and asked me for my suggestions, and I couldn't just hang up on him.

So it should have been no surprise to my friends when I decided to face breast cancer with humor. Read along as I blow up pumpkins, throw eggs, and use my bald head to shame bad drivers. Laugh with me as I thumb my nose at some of cancer's indignities and challenge cancer at every twist and turn of this unpredictable journey called breast cancer. Spoiler alert: if you are the type of person who likes to jump to the end of a book and find out what happens, this line is for you—I survived!

Discovery

Wednesday, September 5, 2012: They say life is a journey. I don't know who "they" are, but I know it is true because I see that phrase so often on coasters, note cards, and signs. My journey started when I found a lump in my breast while I was showering. It scared the bejeebies out of me. I felt the lump, thought, "What is that?" and then felt it again. Everything stopped—time, my breathing, my brain. "Is this something to worry about? Was this there before, and I just didn't feel it? Is this real, or am I overreacting? Is it still there?" I asked myself. I felt again. Yes, it was still there. Crap. When was my last mammogram?

Here is where I tell you that I have a secret weapon: my husband is a general surgeon and has been treating breast cancer for more than twenty years. Over the years, I have noted the changes in my breast texture and location. I have asked him on many occasions to check out a thickening or new texture. All have been normal. When I say that I don't like it, he generally teases me with "Wait till you see what happens next." What? So I determined long ago that I would be a fool not to take advantage of this great resource and have him do my breast exams for me.

When Gene came home that evening, I asked him to check out the lump I had found. He examined me and asked when my next mammogram was due. I told him I was two months past due, so he suggested I call and schedule one. He told me not to get too excited. But he didn't say, "That's nothing," like he had in the past.

The Secret

Monday, September 24: When I found the lump in my breast three weeks ago and set up my mammogram, I thought about calling my mother.

But I held off because we were about to celebrate my parents' fifty-fifth anniversary with a big family reunion at my house. Surely it could wait until after I had a mammogram and knew the results. But my dad died suddenly the day after I found the lump, and everything stopped. I flew to Texas and put everything on hold. Not knowing how long I would be in Texas, I called and rescheduled my mammogram for several weeks later.

So many things were going through my mind as I flew to Texas. I was heartbroken over the loss of my father. I could not imagine being unable to pick up the phone to call him, and yet I was glad he would not be worried about my potential health issues. I wondered if I would be able to travel to Texas in the future to help my mom through dealing with his death. And I wondered if I would be joining him soon.

In the end, I chose not to tell my family anything about my lump while I was there for the funeral. We all had more than we could handle, and why worry about something that none of us could change or do anything about at that point? I embraced my children but didn't tell them either. I looked my family members in the eye and wondered if they would be able to forgive me for not telling them my secret. But I did it out of kindness and to allow them time to grieve for my father. By the time I returned home, I decided not to tell anyone until after the mammogram. After all, I didn't know anything for sure.

The Mammogram

Thursday, September 27: My sweet husband took the day off and came with me to my mammogram appointment. I didn't want to ask him to do this, but it is so nice to have him here. I am nervous. As we sit in the waiting room and wait for the technician to come get me, my leg is tapping as I try to watch whatever is on the waiting-room television. I feel my shoulders tighten up as the minutes drag on. The X-ray tech calls my name, and Gene says, "I'll be right here."

Time to disrobe. "Snaps go in the front," the tech says. A million thoughts are going through my head as I try to concentrate on what the tech is saying. When will someone design a cool-looking cape for women getting mammograms? Or even a warm one? The room is so cold. I feel vulnerable without my bra.

I have been pretty good about getting regular mammograms. I haven't gotten them every year, but overall, I have done pretty well. My last mammogram was fourteen months ago and was normal, so I tell myself not to get too excited. But I know this is different. Deep inside I know that this isn't going to be good news. I think I know what to expect in this mammogram, but I'm about to be surprised.

We take the normal images of both breasts. The tech explains that it is normal to do both breasts even though I felt a lump in only one breast, and I was due for a mammogram anyway. She then explains that we are going to take some more-detailed images. She wasn't kidding. "Detailed images" is medical shorthand for "We are going to squeeze your breasts in so many directions they will resemble Silly Putty when we are done!" As she gets me clamped in for the next set of images, the tech explains that these images are going to be very uncomfortable. I blink. As if the first set weren't already uncomfortable. As she clamps down, she asks, "How are you doing?" I would respond, but I'm pretty sure my lower lip is also clamped in the vise along with my breast, so I can't speak. After several detailed images, she tells me to sit down. The tech is going to talk to the radiologist and see if she wants any other X-rays.

I glance at the wall of various attachments for the mammogram machine. I wonder briefly what they are all for. Unfortunately, I'm about to find out. The tech returns and tells me that we need more images of my right breast and that the radiologist also wants more images of the left breast before we go to sonogram. (Crap! This can't be good.) The tech tells me my husband is in with the radiologist. That really can't be good.

We take close-up images, side images, and I'm squeezed to a point where I can't even whimper when the tech asks if I'm doing okay. She shows me an image of the left breast and points out the calcification they are seeing on the X-rays. It looks like little specks of pepper. There are more specks than I can count quickly, but not thousands. That's not so bad, right? My ears start ringing. I think about asking to sit down, but I don't want to make a scene. I crack jokes with the tech. I am determined to keep up a good front.

The Sonogram

Thursday, September 27: I am lucky that the radiologist is on site and can do my follow-up sonogram immediately. It is a short walk from the mammogram room to the sonogram room. The room is dark, and I joke that I normally take my naps in the afternoon but am willing to make an exception. "Keep breathing," I tell myself. "In and out, one breath at a time." I'm just glad they don't hook me up to a heart monitor, because I can only fake being calm so far.

Warm gel is squirted on my chest and armpit, and we begin. They press firmly on the wand, but it doesn't hurt. I cannot see the screen when they image my right side, but I have a good view for the left side, even though I don't know what I'm looking for. Am I looking for a big white lump? The radiologist explains what we are seeing on the screen and what she is looking for. I play along, but my ears are ringing again. They take a lot of photos and then tell me to get dressed and that they will get my husband

and meet me in the viewing room.

I just want to get this next step over with and get out of the hospital before I fall apart. So, deep breath in and out, I head to the viewing room. I walk in. Everyone looks sympathetic, and the techs all leave the room. I would rather go with them than find out what the radiologist has to say. "Breathe," I tell myself. I glance at the X-ray monitor, and I laugh. The screen saver is an X-ray image of a skeleton holding a microphone. It is hilarious, and I can't help but laugh. Gene walks in, and I glance at him. He steps behind me and squeezes my shoulder. Crap again. Breathe. In and out. One breath at a time.

The radiologist goes through the images, and I nod at all the right moments, but I don't hear very much. I want a backspace key to go back and start my day over. She talks about next steps, and I hear her say that there are three options for biopsy. The words are familiar, but I can't process them. Then she asks what we want to do. I realize I actually have to make a choice, today, when I can't even process what just happened. I glance at Gene, and he says, "We want to go with the stereotactic biopsy." I nod my head. Sounds good to me. No clue what that is, even though the radiologist just explained it. Thank God Gene knows what she is talking about and what to choose. They discuss location and specialist, but I'm no help and leave it to Gene to figure out as I stare at the mammogram images. The radiologist offers to do the biopsy herself or arrange for anyone we choose. I speak up. I have an opinion on this. I ask her to do it. She has been professional and helpful and is willing to work with Gene's schedule. Sold! I'm sticking with you, girlfriend.

I concentrate on getting out of the hospital without blinking. When we get to the parking lot, Gene asks, "How are you doing?" I tell him I'm numb. I keep expecting to cry or shake or react somehow, but I just can't. I start focusing on the words I heard. As we drive home, I ask him to clarify a few things. He has to repeat himself often in the next few days because I just can't seem to connect the dots. Why am I not crying?

The Biopsy

Friday, October 5: You have to have a sense of humor when you walk into a room with a table that has a big hole in the very center, and the tech tells you to climb a ladder and put your right breast in the hole. I look down and say, "But my breast isn't in the center of my body…yet!" The tech, the nurse, and the radiologist all laugh. Seriously, there is no graceful way to do this. I'm laughing because this procedure is so bizarre. They get you centered on the table, lying on your stomach with your breast hanging through the hole. Then they raise the table up to what feels like the ceiling. I glance at the nurse and the ceiling, and I think, "I don't remember her being that tall." It isn't until later that I realize the nurse has climbed a ladder to stand near my head so she can talk to me. And I thought I was uncomfortable! She has to stand there the entire time. I at least get to lie down. The doctor sits on a chair and rolls under the table, and I say, "What are you doing down there?" and we all laugh. I figure if they are entertained, they will work hard to get me a good result.

I get bored easily and find that music relaxes me. So I ask the doctor if I can play my iPod during the biopsy. She explains that I can't wear the headphones while lying on my stomach, but I can place them near my head and turn up the volume. My nurse advocate keeps me entertained by asking about the music I have playing. She notes (well into the procedure) that none of the songs repeat. I explain that I have about four hundred songs on the iPod, and if they start repeating, we have all been there too long.

At some point, the radiologist and tech leave the room to mammogram the samples they have taken. The nurse explains that my breast is still in a clamp and that I have a needle sticking into it, so I should not move. Seriously? Either one of those warnings would have been sufficient. I have a vivid imagination, and I don't like where it is going. What if the doctor decides to go to lunch? What if there is a fire? Is there an emergency release button like at the gas pumps?

After three hours, I'm finally done with the biopsies, and my bra is packed with four ice bags. It is forty-seven degrees outside. This should be fun. The nurse tells me to go out and have a relaxing lunch but that I should change the ice packs every thirty minutes for the next four hours. Yeah, back at you, sweetheart. You have a nice lunch too. At what point during my nice lunch do I pull the ice packs out of my bra and ask the waiter for more ice from the kitchen?

The Witching Hour

Sunday, October 7: I'm not sleeping well. Somewhere between two and four in the morning, I wake up and can't get back to sleep. My brain starts spinning, and a million thoughts go through my head. What can I control? What can't I control? What can I do to get organized (this coming from someone who already has color-coded files and binders for every client and finishes her Christmas shopping in November)? I call this "the witching hour." It is the point where sleep eludes me. My mom and I laugh because she can't sleep either. Since the death of my father last month, she hasn't been sleeping well. We wish we lived closer to each other rather than a thousand miles apart. We come up with codes we could use if we were within sight of each other's house. Porch light on means "I'm up." One flash of the porch light means "Call me." Two flashes mean "Come over." Three flashes mean "Oh crap, I'm busted. Gene is up too."

I think there is going to be a point where I turn into a blubbering idiot and won't be able to stop crying. I woke up about two this morning thinking about it and want to tell Gene that there is going to be a point when I need to cry and that I don't want him to feel like he needs to fix it. Just let me cry. I have images in my head about what my chest is going to look like. Then I just shut it off and tell myself to take one step at a time. But I'm a planner, and I want to know what is coming.

The funny thing is, I would have told you a month ago that I had no emotional attachment to my breasts. I don't think they define me or make me more or less of a woman. I thought that losing a breast or both would be much the same as losing a uterus—one less thing to maintain. But the reality of losing one breast or part of a breast is daunting. It affects the style and size of clothing I can wear. What about symmetry? If I do reconstruction, do I get to pick a size and shape? I don't want to be the same size I am now. I want to be smaller. Does that require surgery on the other side? And let's talk about location. Can I relocate one breast and not the other? Why would I want another saggy breast? I want some lift! But shouldn't they point in the same direction? I laugh at the thought.

Then I back up and tell myself there is still a chance that this may be nothing. I know it isn't a good chance, but I don't skip over that possibility.

The Pathology Report

Monday, October 8: Waiting is awful. It is like being suspended in a place where your feet don't touch the ground and you can't quite reach the ceiling. You can still move your arms and legs, but you don't get anywhere. I had my biopsies on a Friday, so you can just double the normal twenty-four- to forty-eight-hour waiting period to three to four days. People always wonder which is worse, not knowing or hearing bad news. I can assure you that not knowing is worse.

The pathology report is back, and it isn't good. I have invasive ductal carcinoma in multiple areas that is estrogen and progesterone positive and tested positive for the HER2/neu protein. That is doctorspeak for "uh-oh!" Without surgery results, the oncologist would say that I have clinical stage two breast cancer. It sucks to be me!

However, I think we are focusing on the wrong part of the diagnosis. I'm only stage two. I actually laugh as I say this. It could have been far worse. I suspected I was stage one. So stage two is going to be a bit more of a challenge, but I'm focusing on the goal line, which is being cancer-free five years from now.

The Oncologist

Tuesday, October 9: I remember the day the patient packet arrived from the cancer clinic. I thought, "Wait, wait, wait. I haven't even been officially diagnosed with breast cancer. Aren't they jumping the gun?" I opened the packet and read through the materials and filled out the required paperwork.

There is something surreal about driving up to the cancer center. So many thoughts are going through my head: "I don't feel sick. Could this all be a big mistake? Why don't they have an address on the building?" It looks rather nice. I admire the lobby and artwork as we enter. They have free valet parking for patients. Cool!

Gene couldn't go with me, because he had a scheduled procedure on a patient. I don't bat an eye. We have been married for nearly thirty years, and I know the life of a doctor. He would be there if he could, and it is killing him that he can't go with me. But I have asked a friend to go with me who is a nurse, and we will be fine. I glance at my friend Becky, grin, and say, "This is a first for me. Is it also for you?" We laugh. I take her to the best places!

Our escort takes us up to the third floor, where the receptionist gives us a tour of the lobby. As we wait, Becky says, "You are the youngest person here, and the only one with a big smile on her face." Everyone keeps looking at me like I don't get it. I think you choose how you go through life, and I choose to laugh at the hard stuff. It makes me feel better.

I have a wonderful oncologist (if there is such a thing). Dr. Nabi proceeds to draw diagrams; flow charts; and images of my breast, the chemo plan, and the timeline. She even explains all the big words for me. While I may sleep with a doctor, it's not like the Holiday Inn commercial where you develop extraordinary skills because of where you sleep. I build websites. I don't do medicine!

Dr. Nabi explains that I'm going to need surgery and over a year's worth of chemo and radiation. She says that because of my high-risk biopsy results, I get the Cadillac of chemo. "Go big or go home" is my motto! I look her in the eye and say, "You are messing up my travel schedule."

The doctor leaves the room for a few minutes, and Becky and I go into the huddle. You know the huddle. This is where you lean together and talk about all the stuff you don't want to say while the doctor is in the room. Becky says, "Are you thinking what I'm thinking?" I'm sure we are on the same page, so I nod. She says, "This is going to take a lot of energy." Nope. That isn't what I'm thinking. I'm thinking, "I don't have time for this." We laugh. Seriously? Like what I was planning to spend my time on was more important than living?

I Have Breast Cancer

Wednesday, October 10: There. I have said it. I have breast cancer. With just a few days to practice, the words stick in my throat, and my hands shake as I type. It should be easier, but I suspect it is only the first of many hurdles to leap in the next two years. Am I scared? Yes. But I'm also tired and angry, and oddly enough, my sense of humor keeps raising its head and causing my lips to twitch at odd moments. I know this is serious. I get it. But using humor to deal with serious issues has always been easier for me.

The Egg Toss

Friday, October 12: I'm mad. It is four in the morning, and I can't sleep. I'm so tired, and it has been so long since I slept through the night that I want to break something. This is a new feeling for me. I get mad like everyone else, but I remember only one or two times in my life when I wanted to break or kick something. And this is one of them. I look at my cell phone. It looks like a good thing to throw against the wall. But I think better of it. First of all, it would wake Gene up, and that just seems unfair to him. It isn't his fault that I'm mad. Second, I really need my phone to make long-distance calls to my family, so it is going to be inconvenient to be without one. And finally, I can't remember the last time I backed up my phone address book, and it is daunting to think of reentering all that information into a new phone.

I need a plan. I want to break something, but I don't want to clean up the mess. I look around the room for something that will break when I throw it. And then it comes to me. I have a large carton of eggs in the refrigerator. I could take them outside and throw them against a tree, and I wouldn't have to clean up the mess! It turns out that it is only thirty-two degrees outside, and I really don't want to get cold, so I delay my hissy fit and let Gene sleep. I decide to wait to throw the eggs until Gene gets home from work. After all, he might be mad too. I have fifteen eggs, and I want to share the fun. So I spend my time drawing images on the eggs to represent all the things I'm mad at: needles, doctors, pathology reports, Band-Aids and Steri-Strips, cancer, my left breast, my right breast. The list could go on and on, but I have only fifteen eggs, and I'm not a very good artist.

Gene is a good sport. I greet him at the door with a carton of eggs when he returns home, and I say, "Keep your shoes on. I have an activity planned."

He says, "Okay."

Maybe he thinks I have totally lost it, and he is just playing along until the loony van gets here. I don't care. This is going to be cathartic. We march out to the woodpile, and I open the carton and explain what we are going to do. I ask him if he wants the left breast or the right breast. He chuckles and says, "You go first." This man is a saint and knows when not to comment.

I grab one of the eggs and take aim. I bring back my arm and hurl that egg as hard as I can. It actually hurts my arm. I just got my flu shot, and my arm is sore. I miss! Are you kidding me? That isn't cathartic. It just pisses me off! Gene's lips are twitching. "Okay, big guy, you take a turn," I tell him. He hurls his egg and misses too. We need a bigger tree. This just isn't working out like I imagined it. We find a bigger tree, but we miss a lot. No baseball stars in this family. Somewhere in the woods, there are a dozen painted eggs and a happy raccoon.

My husband comes up with a new plan. He tells me that he passed a pumpkin stand on his way home and offers to buy a few pumpkins and let me shoot at them to blow them up. That sounds interesting. Stay tuned for my Annie Oakley story.

I Choose

Friday, October 12: I have always wondered how I would react if I were diagnosed with a life-threatening disease. Would I cry? Would I be calm? Would I be angry? Would I be classy and think of others? Or crawl into a hole and hide? I found out that when given such a diagnosis…I clean out my closet! I'm not kidding. There is stuff in there I wouldn't want my kids to find. So I spend the week sorting, organizing, and finding better hiding places for my stuff.

The thing is, with breast cancer, you don't get diagnosed in one step. It takes multiple steps and multiple doctors before you get confirmation of the disease. So you have a lot of time to think.

I used this time to think and plan. The one thing I have learned already is that you don't have a lot of control over things. My husband has been fantastic. From the first moment, he has told me I'm in charge of this process, and I get to choose how I want to handle it. I get to choose who I tell and when. I get to choose my doctors. I get to choose my treatment plan if there are options. I choose, and he will support me and back me up each step of the way. I love this man and couldn't imagine anyone else at my side.

So I choose to face this illness with humor. I choose to pray for strength. And I choose to put my thoughts on paper and share them with others. It is a coping mechanism for me. It brings clarity. It brings some measure of control. It makes me feel stronger. I choose what I share and what I hide from others. I choose.

Team Kathy

Saturday, October 13: I choose to form a team of people who want to walk beside me and laugh along the way. I'm calling it Team Kathy. Since I'm the self-appointed captain, I want to make sure I have the right people on my team. I want these kinds of people:

- People with positive attitudes
- People who can laugh at themselves and others or at least fake laughing at my humor
- Good fighters
- People with soft shoulders when I need one
- Ironic people
- People who don't understand medical terms
- People who do understand medical terms and can explain them in little words
- People who can say, "Cancer sucks!"
- Creative people
- Skinny and fat people
- Men and women
- People who hate their hair and think going bald might be a good idea
- People who will laugh when I get a Mohawk
- People who will bail me out of jail and not tell Gene if I go a little crazy
- People who will walk beside me

If you have any of these characteristics and think you fit on my team, you are welcome to join me. There are no applications to fill out (though the possibilities intrigue me!) or dues to collect. Just check my blog or drop me an e-mail now and then. Be prepared for a lot of laughs, a few tears, and maybe a cyber pink-pajama party.

The Home Team

Thursday, October 18: This journey would be too difficult if it weren't for my supportive home team—my family. They have supported me over the years through all my bright ideas and antics, which have been just short of getting thrown in jail or doing something in Vegas that had to stay in Vegas (well, there was the one time…).

Gene—my husband and my friend. He laughs with me and at me, which I love. He e-mails me silly things during the day. He has lunch with me. He shows me the world. He is patient and kind. He has answered no less than a thousand of my questions about breast cancer. He calms me when I can't breathe. He holds me when I cry. He knows my fears and insecurities and never tells anyone when I'm bluffing. He can make me smile just by walking into the room. Everything is better when he is at my side.

Nicholas—my oldest child. He is dependable and the first to turn in his vacation homework assignment. (No free rides on our family vacations. Everyone gets an assignment to research our destination and come up with activities and meals for a day.) He visits us often. He talks football and cars with Gene so I don't have to. He finds fixes for my computer when it ticks me off. He asked me to paint stripes in his bathroom—I take that as a compliment and a vote of confidence. He is strong, compassionate, and a gentleman and will be there if I need him.

Steven—my second son. He is my heart, and he inherited my sense of humor. He sees things in the world that the rest of us overlook and points them out to me. He makes me smile and laugh. He never turns in his vacation homework assignment until I threaten him, and I always worry about whether he will show up in the same town the rest of us do on vacation. He has given me the greatest gift for my journey by taking over my business while I'm recovering. When I'm sad, he says, "I love you, Mama."

Danielle—my daughter. People say she is a mini-me, but I see so much more. She is generous, kind, and compassionate. She has grown up so much in the past three years through the deaths of four grandparents. She will make an amazing nurse. She keeps tabs on Gene and me, which makes us laugh. Her smile lights my day. She isn't afraid to do fashion interventions on me, and I will rely on her abilities to teach me 101 ways to tie a scarf around my head when I am bald and to make sure my nail polish matches my shoes.

Sam—my future daughter-in-law. She cruised with us to Alaska this summer and never once tried to push one of us overboard. She always has a smile on her face and a positive attitude. She is caring and kind and fits into our family beautifully. She came to Dad's funeral. She comforts Nick. And she told me that she loved me when I told her my diagnosis. She is family.

And finally, I am blessed with my mother, who I can always talk to; my brother and sister, who are rocks to anchor me; my in-laws and out-laws (you know who you are!), who could not be more supportive; and my many nieces and nephews, who support me. I have the best home-team advantage.

CHAPTER 2
SURGERY

The Surgeon

Thursday, October 11, 2012: On the way to the appointment with the surgeon, Gene asks me if I have decided on what treatment plan I would prefer. Over the past week, he has outlined the available options I will have and answered all my questions. He explains that if I am uncertain or uncomfortable at any point, we can walk out of there without setting a surgery date. I go over my thoughts with him, and he agrees that I have chosen an appropriate plan based on the medical evidence and my comfort zone. We come up with a code phrase I can use if I am uncomfortable or need to think things over. We have tried mind reading in the past, but it has worked with only limited success, so code words are important. My code phrase is "I need to check my calendar."

The surgeon's office is familiar territory. My husband is a surgeon, and I have been walking into surgeons' offices to visit for over twenty years. It gives me confidence to know what to expect. Check in. Fill out paperwork. Have a seat and wait. I hesitate when I have to check the box marked "Cancer" on the registration form. Ugh. That makes it seem real. My heart beats a little faster and my hands shake.

As I sit on the exam table, I glance at Gene sitting on the small bench in the changing area and holding my purse. My lips twitch, and I try not to laugh. I'm not very good at waiting, so I look around the room for something to entertain myself. I see the hand sanitizer, which looks like an upside-down can of whipped cream. I consider squirting it. My husband asks what I'm looking at. I respond, "The flu poster," and my lips twitch again. I'm not sure there is a flu poster in the room, but it is a good bet at this time of year, and he seems to fall for it. I glance at the doctor's stool on wheels and consider sitting on it and spinning around the room, but I'm sure Gene will stop me. I sigh. I fidget.

The surgeon comes in while I'm still fully dressed. I very much appreciate this. To this point, all the doctors have come in to greet me while I'm fully clothed. I wonder if they know how important this is to the patient. It is hard to meet someone for the first time when you are in a paper gown with only your socks on.

I like the surgeon immediately. He talks to me (not my husband) and listens carefully to my responses. I see a hint of sympathy in his eyes when I mention the recent death of my father. He calls me "young." (I now have a doctor's note that says I'm young!) He covers the pathology report with me. The terms are now familiar as I have grilled my poor husband for information for nearly two weeks. He examines me. Once again I am asked to do the Superman pose and put my hands on my hips as the surgeon stares at my chest. I hate this part of the exam, so I occupy myself with deciding what superpowers I would like to have. Probably flight...so I could get the heck out of this room!

We discuss the available options, and the surgeon asks me what I want to do. I consider responding, "Run out of this office and make it all go away," but I know what my options are, and I know what I want. I tell the surgeon that I want to remove the right breast and keep the left breast. He tells me that my plan is exactly what he would recommend, and it reassures me. Gene, my surgeon, and I are all on the same page.

We talk some more and set the surgery date for two weeks from now. I get blood drawn and an EKG. I'm handed more paperwork. We walk out, and I start shaking again. I take deep breaths of air and lean against the car. It is all very real suddenly. But now I have a plan in place, and that gives me some degree of peace.

Etch a Sketch

Monday, October 15: When we left the surgeon's office, I was exhausted. It takes a lot of energy to fake being calm and reasonable. Gene offered to stop and get us drinks on our way home. Unfortunately, he only meant Diet Coke. As he ran into the convenience store, I grabbed the bottle of Tylenol I keep in my purse and got a couple out to swallow with my soft drink. As I looked at the bottle, I noticed instructions on the label that said, "Pull here." So I did. In fact, I pulled the entire label off the bottle. If they only want you to pull it partway, they should be more precise. I tossed the label into the cup holder with some satisfaction.

Gene immediately noticed the label when he got back into the car and asked what it was. I told him I was bored, and the label said, "Pull here," so I did. He responded, "If I had known you were bored, I would have left you with an Etch a Sketch!" That sounded interesting, and I perked up. The best part of an Etch a Sketch is when you are done, you get to shake it and everything disappears. Life should offer an Etch-a-Sketch option. When you make a mistake or don't like what you are seeing, you shake it and it all goes away.

Gene has promised to buy me one for chemotherapy. Those poor nurses at the cancer center have no idea what is coming their way. With my imagination and short attention span, I have trouble sitting idle. Give me fifteen minutes of idle time, and I come up with a project or creative idea that usually causes Gene to groan. How will the nurses put up with me for several hours each week for over a year?

"What Can I Do?"

Tuesday, October 16: I am surrounded by positive and proactive people. The first thing that most of them ask is, "What can I do to help?" This question exhausted me at first, but with the help of a couple of friends, I have come up with a reply.

First and foremost, you can make sure you are current on your mammogram and do self-exams. They work—trust me; I know. Even men can get breast cancer, so they need to check themselves as well. Your health is important to me, and statistically, one in eight women and one in a thousand men will develop breast cancer in her or his lifetime.

You can send me funny or encouraging e-mails and notes in the mail. I will find a basket to collect all of these so I can read them as I go along. Years ago, I created a "Feel Good" file, where I store the many nice notes people have sent me. On days when I wonder if I'm really making a difference in the world, I pull it out and remind myself that I have touched others.

If you live close enough, you can visit or meet me for lunch.

When you see me, you can hug me like you mean it. I don't hurt or feel bad at this time. I feel remarkably good, in fact. I won't break.

You can ask Gene and the kids how they are doing.

You can pray, send positive thoughts, stay positive, and support me as I do this my way.

And finally, if you are so inclined, you can wear something pink for me as a show of support on October 29, my surgery day: nail polish, socks, underwear, shirt, tie, jewelry (oh yes!), or a stinkin' big pink bow in your hair. Send me your photos and make me laugh. (Don't send me photos of your underwear. It would simply be too much to bare!)

The Paperwork

Sunday, October 21: Having surgery requires a lot of paperwork. What happened to electronic medical records? I keep answering the same questions over and over. Maybe it is a test to see if I get the answers right. To test this theory, I change my weight a few pounds every time someone asks me. Not enough to take me back to my twenties, but a pound here and there. So far, none of the doctors' scales match, so why should I stick to one number?

I'm handed a preop folder as I leave the surgeon's office, which I'm told to read over, keep with me at all times, and be sure to bring with me to the hospital. I see that they are assigning some homework: fill out more forms (of course), have my primary care doctor fill out some forms, call the hospital to speak to a registrar who fills out forms, and notify my insurance.

Paperwork—no problem. I'm the queen of paperwork. I will match my paperwork skills with anyone!

Speak to a registrar—I think this translates to "Give the hospital your insurance information." Also no problem. I have this in the bag. I call the very nice lady and respond to a few insurance questions. She asks me if I know where to go on the day of surgery. I tell her that I have no idea. She asks if I have my folder. Of course I do. I'm holding on to it just like I was told to. She instructs me to turn it over and look on the back. There is a giant map on the back with detailed instructions on where to park and where to go. I feel stupid. Who would have thought to look on the back? Then the nurse says, "It looks like I have everything except the type of procedure you will be having." I swallow. I can say this.

"A mastectomy," I reply.

"Oh," she says and pauses. "I'm sorry." This is a great reply. It really is. I mean, what else can a person say? She is very nice and wishes me a speedy recovery. I'm with you, sister!

Notify your insurance—this turns out to be interesting. Basically the same questions are asked, and I roll my eyes at my housekeeper as she passes by and laughs. Then we get to the question I know is coming, and I'm ready for it: "What type of procedure are you having?"

I respond, "A mastectomy." It doesn't get easier, but at least I'm ready for it.

But then I'm thrown a curveball when the lady asks, "And what is that for?"

Seriously? I repeat her question and pause. "Breast cancer?" I reply.

My housekeeper runs for my desk and grabs a note pad and writes, "Tell her you are having a sex-change operation!" I'm laughing so hard at this point that I have to mute the phone. Where are these great lines when I need them?

Roberta's Box

Monday, October 22: Getting a full night's sleep continues to be an issue. There is that moment when I first wake up when hope is eternal, and I hope the first number on the clock is a five or a six. Then I roll over and see a two or a three, and I groan.

I wake in the middle of the night as a million thoughts go through my head. I prepare lists of things to do. I wonder what my head will look like once I'm bald. Will there be divots in it? Do people have to put special products on bald heads to keep them healthy and shiny? What color lipstick goes with a bald head? What will my scar look like? Can I do anything to ease the stress in my family's life? Did I remember to buy dog food?

I mentioned to a friend of mine that I need to find a new way to set aside all of these thoughts and get back to sleep. She told me about what works for her. Years ago, a wise woman named Roberta told her to imagine a box with a lid that locks. When something is keeping you up at night, imagine yourself taking it and putting it into the box and locking the lid. You know it is safe, and it will be there when you can deal with it at a better time. My friend calls this Roberta's Box, and she tells me this imaginary box sits in her closet.

I'm game. I will give it a try. So last night, when I woke up and was worried about all the things I could not control, I imagined a box in my closet. I opened it and put my worries in it. I locked it with a golden key. I rolled over and tried to relax. Then I opened one eye and looked at the clock: 3:15 a.m. *Grrr.* Next time, I'm going to put the clock in the box, and then I can imagine it is whatever time I want it to be.

Waiting

Wednesday, October 24: I have mentioned to several friends that waiting is the hardest part of breast cancer so far. Waiting for the mammogram. Waiting for the biopsy. Waiting for the pathology report. Waiting for the treatment plan. And now, waiting for surgery. I have chosen to look at this two-week period as a gift. Not everyone gets the luxury of time when their life is about to change. I have two weeks to pester the dickens out of my family and friends!

In true Kathy style, I have gone into overdrive in organizing my house. My office would bring a tear to Martha Stewart's eye. I have cleaned out my closet and (gasp) even labeled the boxes on the shelves. I have done my fall pickup outside and created a list for Dean (our handyman) to do over the next month. I have arranged backup snow removal in case I can't do it. I have lists and lists of things to do or tell other people to do. And I have even purchased more than half of the things on my Christmas list *and* wrapped them! When I walked to the door of our storage room this weekend, my husband said, "*No!* Don't even think about it. There is no way you can organize and get that finished in time, and you are going to leave me a big mess." So I followed him out to his workshop on Monday to see what he was working on. He saw me glancing around and the wheels in my brain turning. "*No*," he said.

I think my friends have gotten together to find some form of distraction. We had a delightful dinner with friends on Monday night and talked about travel and kids and normal things. On Tuesday, my friend Joanne treated me to an "all about me" day. We went to a spa and had our first-ever facials. Trudie, my new best friend, did things to my face that put me in a state of bliss. She buffed, polished, steamed, and toned me to the point where my face is smoother than it was when I was nine years old. Joanne and I left the spa, and all we could say was, "Oh man. We have to do that again." We had lunch, and I rounded out the afternoon with a nap. Later in the week, Gene and I met friends who drove two hours to have dinner with us, and we laughed and talked and had such a great time. I smiled at Gene and held his hand on the drive home and said, "I had such a great day."

I feel strong. I feel the support of my friends and family. I can't wait for my mom to arrive on Saturday. I feel ready for surgery. Bring it on! Shoot, I have to wait until Monday for surgery.

Surgery Morning

Monday, October 29: I have received so many cards, messages, prayers, and gifts and feel humbled and supported by all of you. I have laughed at your messages and cried at your notes. I had a good week, and I'm ready for surgery. My mom has arrived, and moms always make things better. She came bearing gifts from my relatives and arms full of love. I have prayer blankets and feel wrapped in their warmth.

The final step before surgery was to remove my toenail polish, and I find that I have a bit of a rebel in me. I asked my husband if there was any medical reason for me to do this, and he told me to just follow the instructions. Well, I plan to fight breast cancer…and fight to change stupid rules! So I left the nail polish on my middle toes as an act of rebellion. I have pink socks on, so maybe they won't notice. I will remove my jewelry, but only because I happen to love it and want it safe. I will follow the instructions and not shave my right armpit—but I will shave the other one! I will not eat or drink anything after midnight, but someone better wave a cup of coffee under my nose about seven o'clock or dye the IV solution coffee color. I will laugh if they mark "noncompliant patient" on my chart.

I know I have the easy part today as I get to sleep through the procedure. I know how hard waiting is, so I will have Steven post a quick update on my blog sometime late tonight when he gets to the house. Don't forget to send me your photos if you are wearing pink!

The Surgery

Monday, October 29: We arrive at the hospital promptly at 8:30 a.m. and are immediately escorted back to a preop room. After I change into my couture backless gown and robe, Gene, my mom, and Danielle are allowed to spend the morning with me. I have put on the gown and robe that are given to me, but I refuse to wear the hospital socks. I have nice, new pink socks—a gift from my niece and nephew—and they are way cuter than the hospital socks. The day starts well with this strike for independence.

I am surprisingly calm and keep expecting to get nervous or upset, but I think that mentally, I am just plain ready to get the surgery over with. I laugh and chat with my family, and they all roll their eyes when I say I am bored. A numbing cream is applied to my breast to help with the upcoming lymph node injections.

At ten o'clock, I am taken up to radiology to get radioactive dye injected into my breast to help identify the sentinel lymph node for biopsy. This is a process that I am worried about because I have heard that it is quite painful. Dr. Hemann is my radiologist once again. She just can't seem to get enough of me! She has been with me for the initial mammogram, sonogram, and biopsy. We laugh and joke a bit, and she explains the process. She even comments to Gene that I'm a compliant patient. I'm hoping she doesn't lift the sheet and see my pink socks, not to mention the nail polish on my middle toes!

Dr. Hemann explains that the injection will sting a lot, but it fades quickly (within a minute). I take a few deep breaths and tell her to go for it. The nurse offers to hold my hand, but I decline and consider asking for a bullet. The injection really stings, but I must say that in the scheme of things, it isn't that bad. By no means is it the worst thing I have had done. The radiologist then takes a marker and circles the injection site, writes the date and time, and puts her initials. When we get back to the preop room, I tell my mom that I now have an expiration date on my right breast.

As they wheel me back to my preop room, we pass the cafeteria. I'm hungry, really hungry, and I try to read the sign to see what the soup specials are for today. I pass a large cart stacked high with plastic containers holding sandwiches and cantaloupe. I like sandwiches. I like cantaloupe. I am parked next to the food cart as we wait for the elevator. Gene laughs and says, "This is cruel."

Now I need to wait two hours for the radioactive dye to work. At half past eleven, I start to get a little anxious. This is really happening. The anesthesiologist asks if I would like something to calm me. You betcha!

Don't hold back on the drugs. Give me anything you have in that little bag of yours. About ten minutes before noon, two nurses come in and give me half of an injection and tell my family to say their good-byes. I want to tell my mom to take care of Gene if something goes wrong, but I can't get the words out. We hug. I expect to cry but I don't. I tell them I'm okay, and I really mean it.

I remember going into the OR and moving to the operating table. Things look familiar…and that pretty much ends my day. I wake up in recovery and feel some pain, but not a lot. I'm very, very tired and can't figure out where I am. Things start to make sense, and I want to ask them to bring my husband back. I have questions for him that I'm not sure the nurse will be allowed to answer, and I know he will tell me the truth. After an hour, the nurses roll me through the labyrinth of hallways, and then I see Gene. I manage to wait until I get to my room before asking about the sentinel (lymph) node. He tells me it is clear. I breathe a big sigh of relief.

Successful Surgery!

Monday, October 29: Mom wanted me to get online after she came out of recovery to let everyone know that she is well and everything went well in surgery. Apologies for the late update. (She just said *after* surgery, not *right after!*) We visited her in the hospital, and she was in good spirits, a little worn out and ready for some well-deserved rest, but doing very well. Thank you all so much for the flowers and well wishes. Knowing Mom, she will be up and writing again in no time!

—Steven

The Room

Tuesday, October 30: My room at the hospital was quite nice. First of all, there were flowers in it, and I think flowers make any room nicer. It also came complete with a DVD player, Internet hookups, and a sofa that pulled out to form a bed. For some reason, Gene wouldn't give me my cell phone or laptop. He seems to think that things that seem like a good idea after surgery usually aren't.

A few years ago, after I had surgery, Gene went to fill my pain meds and left my cell phone within reach. It suddenly seemed very important for me to call my friend Tess so she could hear my voice. I knew (or thought I knew) she was waiting anxiously to hear from me personally. So I called her. I can still hear her laughing and asking, "Where is Gene?"

So I decided to let Gene be in charge of electronic devices this time. It was just too hard to keep my eyes open. I do remember Danielle showing me dozens of photos of friends and family wearing pink. I kept saying,

"Who is that? I don't know them," or "Aw, that is so sweet."

Danielle would patiently reply, "Mom, you do know them. They have your cell phone number."

I had a very nice view of an ENT (ear, nose, and throat) building. I know this because as I got up to go to the bathroom in my backless gown, dragging my IV pole, I realized I was mooning them. At one point, I turned to Gene and said, "It serves them right. It's about time they see a few butts." Where do these thoughts come from? I'm blaming the anesthesia.

I'm Back!

Wednesday, October 31: It is a beautiful, sunny Halloween day, and I'm dressed up as a breast cancer survivor—pink socks, gray shawl, prayer blanket! I had a decent night last night but was so grateful to be in my own bed that I would have taken any amount of discomfort just to get home. It took us until five to get home yesterday, and I thought I would go nuts before we got out of the hospital. A friend had dinner waiting for us.

I'm not having a lot of pain today but having to take some pain pills due to drain issues. So nice to have Mom, Steven, and Danielle around today to deal with deliveries, refrigerator repairs, dry cleaners, and so on. Steven and Mom are working on dinner, and I'm laughing as they try to find things in my kitchen. I spent most of the day chatting with Mom and Steven and watching old movies. Computer work is going to have to wait another day or two due to swelling under my right arm and side. And that drain is most inconvenient. But all in all, much better than anticipated, so all is good. I am surprised at how calm I was on Monday. I'm glad to have this step behind me. Thank you all so much for your prayers and support. It means so much to me.

Sleep

Thursday, November 1: Isn't it amazing the difference a little sleep can bring? Just prior to surgery, a breast cancer survivor sent me an e-mail telling me to make sure I had lots of pillows. I happen to be a person who regularly purchases new pillows in search of the perfect pillow, so I thought I was set. It turns out that there are not enough pillows in the universe to get comfortable in bed the first few nights after surgery.

When I first came home from the hospital, I knew that getting comfortable in bed might be a problem. But it had to be better than the hospital, right? What I didn't anticipate was how restricted my sleeping positions would be. I couldn't sleep on my left side, because the port area (near my shoulder) was incredibly tender. I couldn't sleep on my right side, because the drain was in the way and the suture area under my arm was sore. I had to sleep on my back. I tossed, I sighed, I whimpered, and I finally got up around four in the morning to rest in the chair.

On my second night home, I decided there had to be a better solution. I created a cocoon of pillows and tried to crawl into the hollow. Pillows under my arms, pillows under my knees, pillows everywhere. It was incredibly comfortable for about two minutes. Then I realized why those silkworms always morph into moths. It is in order to get out of that constricting cocoon! Back to the chair I go.

The one bright spot in these sleepless mornings was the opportunity to have long talks with my mother. She hasn't been sleeping either since the death of my father six weeks ago. So we set up a system. When I got up between two and four, I would turn on the lights to the basement stairway. If she woke up and saw the lights, she would come up and talk to me. We spent hours talking during the week of her visit. We talked about our fears and frustrations. We talked about our crazy relatives and our perfect dogs. We talked about breast cancer and death and hope and survival. I would gladly give up sleep to have these conversations again.

Now that a few days have passed, sleep is becoming a bit easier. Some nights I sleep five or six hours; some nights I get only a few hours of sleep. But I have stopped measuring the nights by the number of hours and more by how I feel when I wake up. I suspect that I will have plenty of time to sleep during chemo.

The Wound

Thursday, November 1: I have read my share of books and watched enough Lifetime Channel movies to know that many women are afraid to look at the scars on their chests after surgery. For me, the unknown has always been more frightening than the known. So when my mom asked me what I felt when I looked at my scar, my lips twitched, and I said, "It sure beats dying!" I don't want to downplay what others feel. This is just my personal reaction.

I didn't get to see the scar all at once. It came in stages. I woke up in recovery, and when I could finally keep my eyes open for a few minutes at a time, I couldn't help but glance down and notice the change in my bustline. Because the left breast was not removed, it gave the appearance that the right side was actually concave, and this threw me for a minute. I was also reassured because the left breast was still there. You see, when I first started waking up, I felt some stinging on the left side. In my confused state, I wondered if the lymph nodes had been involved and if they felt they should go ahead and take the left breast as well. As it turns out, the stinging I felt was the port the surgeon inserted so that chemo will be easier.

Most of that night was spent dozing in and out of sleep. The next morning, I decided to take a peek and see what the surgery site looked like. The incision was covered in gauze and had a drain line coming from it. It didn't look as smooth as I thought it would, but there wasn't much to see. Later in the day, the surgeon came in and removed the dressing. Yes, I peeked. Like I said, I would rather know than not know.

Well, it doesn't look like I thought it would, and the incision is much longer than I expected. Some of the irregularity is probably due to swelling. The line isn't straight but curves downward under my armpit. Not being an expert in the field, I suspect that some of this is due to my particular anatomy and size and that incisions can vary from patient to patient.

So back to Mom's question: What do I feel? Truly, the first thought I had was, "I can live with this." I don't feel emotional or frightened by it. I don't feel less of a woman. I don't feel embarrassed by the lack of a breast when I go out. I feel like it is part of a process to stay alive, and I want to live. I would much rather lose some breast tissue than risk losing my life. I was so surprised by the roller coaster of emotions prior to surgery, and I find that being on this side of surgery is so much better.

On the other hand, I do find the issue of my left breast hanging out and being unsupported to be problematic. It is one thing for it to hang out when my mom and husband are around, but another thing entirely when my sons are visiting. Don't get me wrong, my sons are great. It is a mom thing. Seriously, I have said the word "breast" to my grown sons so many times in the past few weeks, and I cringe each time. I told my mom that I had considered using a bandanna to make a sling for my left breast but that I was afraid it would hurt if I tried to tie the sling around my neck. We laughed and laughed.

The Surgery Pathology Report

Monday, November 5: Late Friday, I received a call from the surgeon's office regarding my surgery pathology report. It contained very good news. The nurse told me the surgeon had not seen the report yet, but she could give me a quick summary. The two key pieces were that the margins were clear and that there were no signs of cancer in the sentinel node. The surgeon will cover the complete report with me when I see him in ten days.

For those who don't speak doctor, a simplistic explanation would be as follows: Margins are the outside edges of the tissue that they removed. They look for any stray cells of cancer that may be outside of the primary tumor area. If the margins are clear, people tend to say, "They got it all." If they find stray cells, further surgery or treatment is required.

As for the sentinel node, it is the first lymph node that filters from the breast. So it would be the first node that cancer reaches. Radioactive dye is injected into the breast, and the surgeon looks for the first node (or nodes) the dye reaches. This is the sentinel node, and the most likely place to have cancer if cancer has spread to the lymph nodes. If this node is clean, it is likely that all other nodes are as well.

There are other pathology details still to be explored, but this was wonderful news to receive on Friday. I meet with the oncologist this week to set a chemo schedule, but I feel that I have already won part of the battle.

Reality

Monday, November 5: My company has left, and it is back to reality. I find myself lying in bed and wondering, "Why get up?" Who will fill my water glass when it is half-empty? Who will spoil Gene by preparing his breakfast every morning? Who will load the dishwasher and do the list of honey-dos? Yes, I will admit that I saw an opportunity and jumped on it. I prepared a list of odd jobs that I didn't want to do and had my kids do them while they were here (snicker). The firewood rack is loaded, the garden shovels have been replaced by snow shovels, the bird feeders have been put away for the winter, and the garage has been blown out. My children even stripped their beds and washed and replaced the sheets before they left. You don't get opportunities like this every day!

Tomorrow promises to be a hilarious day. I am going wig shopping with my hairstylist and my friends Becky and Tess. I plan to experiment with some new looks as well as some color changes until I find the "new me." Then we plan to go to lunch and finish off the afternoon at our favorite jewelry store. Short of having a facial and pedicure, this is the perfect day.

The Terrible Patient

Tuesday, November 6: I'm a terrible patient. It is probably because I have no patience. I expect more out of myself than I expect out of others, and I tend to push myself to unrealistic limits. The list of things I have done since surgery (while I'm supposed to be recovering) borders on the line between inadvisable and "Are you out of your mind?" And the result is that "reason" came and clubbed me over the head last night.

By six o'clock, I could hardly lift my arms. This could be due in part to my overenthusiastic exercise routine. The nice physical therapist visited me in the hospital with a list of exercises I should do in recovery. I am to do only one exercise, twice a day, until the drain comes out. Well, my shoulder is stiff and weak, so I figured, why do two sets when I could do, let's say for argument, six or more sets? I also used that arm to reorganize my pantry (like someone is going to come in and grade it?) and move some laundry. Then it seemed like a good idea to take Dolly Dog out for a couple of walks. I'm really sorry we have put the chairs away for the winter, because I could have used one about halfway back to the house.

I was very thankful that a neighbor had dropped some chili off so I didn't have to actually cook dinner. I spent the rest of the evening complaining that my back, shoulder, side, arm, neck, and everything else hurt. I woke up this morning feeling like I had been drugged and simply wanted to pull the covers over my head. Lesson learned...for the moment.

Drains

Tuesday, November 6: My biggest issue with surgery is the drain line. It has become an unwelcome, constant companion, and I blame everything on the drain. I cannot wait to have it removed. I would lie and try to get it out early, but Gene assures me that I really don't want to take it out too soon. So I continue to take care of this nuisance much like a high school student takes care of a pretend egg baby.

Why do I hate it? Let me count the ways:

1. It gets in the way when I shower. I have resolved this issue by wearing a name-badge lanyard while I shower and clipping it to the drain bulb.
2. It is disgusting looking. The tube is always hanging out, even when I slip it into the convenient pocket in my "free" camisole the hospital "gave" me. The camisole has a long pocket that resembles a muffler across the belly. So when I put the drain bulb in it, it puts a hump in front of my belly button that looks like my boob has fallen.
3. It makes it impossible to sleep on my right side. And my left side hurts because the port is still healing. So that leaves sleeping on my back.
4. Gross stuff comes out of it, and I have to measure the gross stuff.

Thank-You Notes

Wednesday, November 7: What is the punishment for not getting your thank-you notes out on time? I ask this because I am so far behind on sending thank-you notes. I grew up in the South, where there is an etiquette for all things, and the first etiquette rule in any book is "Send a handwritten thank-you within one week of receiving a gift." I'm pretty sure it is carved into a great stone in the South somewhere. I know this is true because my mother taught it to me. I continue to write thank-you notes promptly to this day, because I know my mother is quite capable of driving up from Texas and reminding me of my duty. Friends have even commented that my thank-you notes often beat them home.

So what to do with this growing list of unwritten thank-you notes? First of all, if you have dropped off, mailed, or sent anything to the hospital or otherwise supported me, thank you. This by no means excuses me from writing the notes. I know my duty. Trust me, my mom will call you if you try to give me a pass. Mom did tell me once that there are extensions to the one-week rule in the case of grief or immobility. I'm not immobile, but I do have breast cancer—or at least I did a week ago. Do you think this qualifies for an extension?

In the meantime, please accept my heartfelt thank-you for all the support you have shown through my diagnosis and surgery.

The Wandering Breast

Thursday, November 8: There are a few things the doctors and survivors don't tell you about before surgery, one of which is the wandering breast. Since I had only one breast removed, and I cannot wear a bra until my incision heals, that leaves my left breast free to do its own thing. And right now, it seems a bit lost. I told my husband that I'm annoyed that my breast wants to take up residence under my armpit.

Prior to surgery, there was balance in my life. The two girls hung out together and learned to share space. They even supported each other now and then. When I slept, they were pillow buddies and would rest on each other while I slept on my side. Now I find the left breast wandering as I toss and turn in search of a comfortable position to sleep. It is amazing how far it can travel.

I'm reminded of the old Carol Burnett comedy sketches where one of the guest stars would be dressed as a woman. Inevitably during the skit, his oranges would relocate, and one would be under the armpit while the other would be up on the shoulder. There would be an adjustment, and all the characters would die laughing. Well, I'm certainly finding my own humor.

I told my husband that I'm considering saving some money and just stuffing socks into the empty bra pocket when I can finally wear a bra again. "It worked when I was thirteen," I told him, "so it should certainly work now."

Without blinking, he responded, "Then you better plan on buying a lot of lead shot if you want it to look like the other side." I can't help it. That is funny!

The Prayer Quilt

Friday, November 9: My niece is a youth minister in Texas, and her church creates prayer quilts for people going through difficult times. The workers pray as they sew the quilts. When they finish a quilt, they tie yarn to it and leave the strands long. The quilt is passed around, and each person ties a knot as they pray for you.

This quilt was passed around my family and their friends in Texas and even taken to a Race for the Cure in Dallas/Fort Worth. Complete strangers have heard my story and prayed for me. There are dozens and dozens of knots tied in the yarn. This touches me profoundly. I try to tell people about the quilt but find that it brings me to tears each time, and I cannot finish the sentence. I am so completely moved by the outpouring of support during this difficult journey.

I have been added to so many prayer chains and individual prayers this past month. I cannot express how much it means to me when someone says they will be praying for me. I have a deep faith in God and know that he walks with me on this journey and carries me when the journey is too difficult. And I very much believe in the power of prayer.

If a life is measured by the number of people you touch in your lifetime, then I hope each of you know that you are a superstar.

CHAPTER 3
CHEMOTHERAPY PHASE ONE

Chemo or No Chemo?

Thursday, November 8, 2012: Several people have asked my why I'm having chemo if "they got it all," so I thought I would try to explain. Physicians treating cancer don't say "we got it all." Instead they talk about lymph nodes and clear margins (see the pathology report posting in chapter 2). But most of us simplify the results by saying, "They got it all." Unfortunately, cancer is a sneaky little devil and can be unpredictable. Physicians and researchers continue to study it and predict its behavior and treat patients accordingly.

My physicians have taken my pathology report, family history, age, and other factors into consideration and have determined that their goal is to give me the best possible chance to reach my eightieth birthday and beyond, and that means chemo and radiation therapy for over a year. Since I am considered young (yes, I have a doctor's note to prove it) and my cancer is aggressive, chemo ensures my best chance of survival.

The second question that I'm getting a lot is "Why are you getting chemo for over a year?" According to my pathology report, I tested HER2/neu positive in each of the tumor areas. What this means is that my cancer is faster growing and more aggressive than some other breast cancers. My research says that only 25 percent of all breast cancers test positive for HER2/neu. So the doctors want to make sure that any traces of cancer are eliminated by using a very targeted therapy that lasts over a year. The good news is that there is a targeted treatment for my type of cancer.

There are many, many protocols for chemo; and mine is just one of them, and it happens to be an extensive and long treatment. But I'm going to take it one step at a time and set goals for each step.

Chemo Schedule

Saturday, November 10: My first chemo is scheduled for next Wednesday, and then there are three more Wednesdays (every other), with phase one ending on December 26. Because of my diagnosis, I am on an accelerated schedule with chemo every two weeks rather than every three weeks. My doctor has explained that phase one of chemo is a roller coaster of feeling great on chemo day, followed by a downward slope to day seven, which is awful, followed by an upward slope to feeling good again on day fourteen, at which point we start all over. So it looks like Thanksgiving week will be icky for me. Danielle is going to sit with me on my first chemo morning until she has to go to clinic. I'm so fortunate that she is doing her clinical rotation at the hospital next to the cancer center. The doctor assured me that I will feel fine after chemo and will be able to drive myself home. The side effects for phase one include:

- Fatigue
- Hair loss
- Nausea/vomiting
- Increased risk of infection
- Anemia
- Increased risk of bleeding
- Heart dysfunction
- Mouth sores

We like to call phase one the really, really bad stuff. The good news is that there are only four infusions in phase one. I'm going to have to come up with a fun scale to represent my progress. My hair should fall out within ten days and be gone by Thanksgiving weekend. I'm not looking forward to losing my hair.

Phase two (known as the really bad stuff) is twelve weeks long and given weekly and will start in January. Phase three (known as the not-so-bad stuff) will last thirty-two weeks but will be given only every three weeks. I find the schedule daunting if I look at it as a whole, but when you break it into smaller pieces…it just sucks!

Meet Raquel

Wednesday, November 14: On Monday, I went wig shopping with Gene, Danielle, and Shawn (my amazing hairstylist), and it wasn't as fun as I had anticipated. I thought we would go to a wig shop where there would be lots of wigs, and I would try them on and then maybe have to order a different color. Not so much. There were five wigs on the wall, and all looked a bit…sad. The lady handed us about six catalogues to look through and dozens of hair samples to match to my hair.

I readjusted my thinking and started flipping through the books, and then I froze. My brain said, "This is too hard." I whispered to Shawn, "Help me." I could tell by his face that he knew I wasn't joking around. I kept a smile on my face and tried to make jokes, but everything was falling flat. Thank God Gene was there. While the rest of us were looking a little lost, Gene promptly picked out two styles of wigs, and Shawn loved them and agreed that they were similar to my current cut. I simply couldn't process the idea.

Part of the problem in picking out a style for me is that the model for all of the wigs in the catalogue was Raquel Welch. On my best day, I don't resemble Raquel, and I don't have auburn hair. So putting my face under her auburn hair just didn't click for me. I'm pretty sure she looks good in anything. I just couldn't visualize myself in any of the wigs.

Shawn and Danielle were able to color-match my hair pretty well, so that part was easy. Danielle and Gene were great at deciding on the fine details and ordering the wig for me. I had a great team with me. I did manage to get out of there without crying but had tears streaming down my face when we got in the car. Fortunately, only Gene was with me at that point. He gets all the awful jobs.

On the upside, we decided to turn this appointment around and do something truly fun. For the past ten or so years, I have admired a glass head in Shawn's hair salon. It makes me smile every time I see it. I figure, why buy a Styrofoam wig stand at forty-five dollars or more when I can get a decorator piece for nineteen dollars! So we went to Pier 1 and purchased a glass head to use as a wig stand. It is a bottle-green glass head that is hollow. It has the advantage of being heavy, so it won't fall over in the night. Can you imagine how freaked Dolly Dog would be if my head fell over and the wig hit the floor next to her? She might never recover!

The saleslady carefully wrapped the glass head in tissue paper, and we left with our purchase. I smiled as Gene walked through the parking lot swinging the bag. He gently placed it in the backseat, and I snickered. As soon as he turned the first corner, it started rolling around the backseat. Gene said, "Don't lose your head," and we laughed. It continued to roll until I reached around and tossed my purse on top of it. When we got home, Gene said, "I've got your head." If only it were true!

I told Gene that we needed to name it if it was going to be sleeping in the same room with us. When the Vinton Breast Cancer Survivors group dropped off a care package that included a stocking cap, I couldn't resist putting it on the glass head. And then it came to me. From that moment on, she would be known as Raquel.

First Day of Chemo

Thursday, November 15: I have been trying to decide what to say about my very, very long first day of chemo. I arrived at nine o'clock and left at two thirty. Danielle was able to be with me the entire time. Her supervisor allowed her to take a few hours off so that she could finish treatment with me. We managed to play nice with everyone since it was my first day. Actually, Danielle played nice and listened to all the instructions. I, on the other hand, zoned out at some point and resorted to just smiling and nodding. I was in information overload.

I had so many visitors—social services, nutrition, patient relations, and on and on. I pretty much tuned people out until I heard the word "massage," and then I perked up and said, "Heck yes, I want one!" And each person had a business card and printed materials to go along with their talk. I'm going to have to buy a special business card holder for all my physician cards and cancer center cards. And as Gene said, I'm going to need a bigger folder for breast cancer.

We had a lovely private chemo room with a window, and the chair had seat heaters and vibrators! You can't hardly beat that. And there was a snack lady. About once an hour, she came around with a basket of goodies to tempt and treat me. All those forbidden snacks over the years were in one handy basket that came waving in front of me. It was just too much! One of my trigger foods that I don't allow in the house is Chex Mix, because I just can't stop eating it. And there it sat, in not one but two flavors in the basket. And they were free! Is this heaven? Nope, still chemo, but it comes with perks. I sipped and snacked for five hours. Oddly enough, the thing that tasted the best was the little container of cottage cheese that I shared with Danielle. (By the way, visitors get access to the snack basket as well. Oh boy! Wait till I tell Gene.)

Chemo starts with all the premeds: antinausea and so on. Chemo premeds are the various medications given to me to help reduce the side effects of chemotherapy. It seems like there are dozens of IV bags, and some drip for ten minutes, some five minutes, and the last one is an hour. And then there is the "direct push" chemo meds that come in a hazardous materials bag. I have to say, it took everything in me to sit still and not panic when that medicine was given to me. For heaven's sake, it says "Hazardous Material" on the bag, and they want to put it in my IV?

During one infusion, I was instructed to eat ice chips or a Popsicle during the infusion. This particular chemo medication attacks soft tissue, and the nurses wanted to protect my gums, cheeks, and tongue. Studies have determined that sucking on ice chips or cold products help reduce the damage to those soft tissues because the cold ice slows the blood flow to these tissues. I chomped on my Popsicle like my life depended on it.

The day was long, but I survived my first chemo and was able to drive myself home. I'm now 25 percent done with phase one.

Raquel Goes AWOL

Sunday, November 18: When I ordered my wig on Monday, I was told that it would be overnight shipped and should arrive either Tuesday or Wednesday and the salon would call me. When I did not hear from them by Friday, I called to see if the wig had arrived. When no one could find the wig, I decided to name my wig Raquel on good days and Rachel on her rebellious days.

For several years, a group of us used to travel to meetings in Chicago. Occasionally, we would take a friend of ours named Gretchen with us. Inexplicably, when we got to Chicago, people would start to call her Rachel instead of Gretchen. We don't know why. Maybe she looked like a Rachel, but we all knew her name was Gretchen. So we decided to have some fun with it, and Rachel became Gretchen's alter ego. Shouldn't my wig have an alter ego as well?

After a bit of detective work, Rachel (the wig) was found, and I set up an appointment to pick her up. I took Gene along to read the rules to her. It is difficult enough to find my car keys on any given day. I don't need to be searching for my wig! But I'm sorry. she is going to have to ride in the backseat on the way home.

When I sat in the chair and the stylist put the wig on, I had to look away. It did not look like my hair, nor was the cut or texture similar to my style. I glanced back at the mirror, and I saw a sad old woman. It was hard to face. The stylist kept talking and working with the wig, and it became better, bit by bit. I refused to cry. I glanced at my husband, and he didn't look horrified. I asked him what he thought, and he responded, "It looks nice and like real hair." I couldn't decide if he was out of his mind or if he was being incredibly kind. I took another look in the mirror, and the wig wasn't so bad. But it wasn't me.

Now is the time when I need to repeat to myself that this is only temporary. My hair doesn't define me. Cancer doesn't define me. My heart and what I do with my life define me. And if I can laugh this off, I am well on my way to a cure.

So come on, Raquel. Please have more good days than bad. And on the Rachel days, I will always have Gretchen, Tess, Barb, and all my friends with me and the memories of fun times in Chicago!

Blowing Up Pumpkins—25 Percent Done!

Sunday, November 18: Blowing up a pumpkin is therapeutic—I don't care who you are. It makes me laugh. While I find a year of chemo daunting, it does give me many opportunities to have some fun. Phase one, the super-sucky phase, requires some form of therapy to mark the passing of each of the four chemo sessions. So I have chosen to blow up pumpkins.

Since it gets dark about five o'clock in Iowa this time of year, it was too late on Wednesday to take care of the task. So we gathered our gear and headed down to the pond to take care of business this afternoon. It was a beautiful day. I fed the fish in the pond in hopes of pacifying them before the fireworks began. We placed the pumpkin on a tree stump, and we mixed the Tannerite.

Tannerite tends to be a bit harder to blow up than the package states, but we were being cautious and following the rules. We set the target on the stem of the pumpkin, aimed, fired…and blew the target off the pumpkin and harmlessly into the water. The pumpkin continued to sit nicely on the stump without injury. It seems to me that blowing off steam is a lot harder in practice than in theory.

We continued to blow all kinds of holes in the pumpkin with no explosion, until Gene got just the right hit and *POW!* A big, orange ball of flame exploded the pumpkin. My mouth was a big *O*, and my eyes were huge, and then I doubled over laughing. But there was still some pumpkin left, so we added more targets and started shooting until the second explosion. A large cloud of smoke came our way, and I was laughing so hard that I was gasping. Pieces of pumpkin were flying into the pond, and I wondered what the fish were thinking. I also wondered what the neighbors were thinking.

Yes, blowing up pumpkins is therapeutic—I don't care who you are.

The Big Reveal

Thursday, November 22: Go ahead. Admit it. You have always wondered what your head would look like shaved. I know I have. Not that I have ever been tempted to shave my head. Would my scalp be nice and smooth or have divots or lumps? Are there any old childhood scars from the jungle gym or swings? Birthmarks? Moles? It is a mystery, especially if you are like me and have nice, thick hair. As it turns out, I have a nice, smooth head.

I decided to go proactive and shave my head before my hair fell out from chemo. I didn't want the memory of handfuls of hair falling out over Thanksgiving, so I set up an appointment to shave my head on my schedule. Take that, cancer! You aren't in charge of me!

So off to Shawn's we went to get my new do. We were jacked up on coffee and Diet Coke—it pays to be fortified when one goes through these experiences. We entered D'aversa Salon an hour before they opened. I took part of my number-one support team of family and friends as backup: Tess—the little voice that whispers in my ear, "Oh, go ahead and do it. I'm an attorney, and I can talk us out of trouble." Becky—the voice of reason but who will support me if I decide to listen to Tess.

Danielle—number-one camera operator and the one who occasionally says, "No, Mom. That isn't a good idea." And Shawn—number-one hairstylist and friend who is always good for a laugh and a hug.

I told Becky to just walk in and listen for the laughter and she would find us. Sure enough, that is all it took. Shawn didn't waste any time. He said, "Ready?" and took a big swipe. That's when I told him I had changed my mind. He didn't even blink. He knows me well and said, "Too late!" and kept going. So I asked for a Mohawk. Seriously, how often do you get to do that in your life? Shawn not only gave me a Mohawk but also the Kewpie-doll curl in front for a short time. We played. We laughed. We took pictures. We had fun.

I thought shaving my head would be hard. I thought I might cry. But it was really funny. At one point, I tried to squeak out a tear, sniffed, and said, "You know what would make me feel better? If all of you would shave your heads in support." Nope. No takers. Only Shawn is a true friend. But then, he already shaves his head.

The Big Reveal II

Saturday, November 24: It has taken me a few days to get the nerve up to float some photos of the big reveal (head shave) on my blog and on Facebook. I must say that everyone was very kind in their comments. My cousin Phillip said he thought I had sent him photos of Sinead O'Connor for a second. I can see his confusion!

I have to tell you that several survivors told me I would feel better once I shaved my head. And they were right. The fear of the unknown is much worse than the actual process, in my opinion. Shawn was a wonderful friend and hairstylist and helped tremendously. I laughed until my sides hurt. My friends were very supportive, if not enjoying themselves a bit too much! And everyone has been kind about the result. But hey, I'm fighting for my life, so what is a little hair between friends? And I have to say, when the chin and upper lip hairs fell out this morning, I grinned! Nobody talks about those little devils, but I will not miss them!

The Holiday Season

Sunday, November 25: I love the holidays. Ask anybody. I have a permanent smile plastered on my face beginning November 1 and ending after New Year's. I love the weather—cool, crisp mornings with changing leaves. I love the food. I love buying presents. I'm that obnoxious person who has her shopping done by Thanksgiving and laughs at the people who actually go out on Black Friday. I, by contrast, use that time to put up my beautiful Christmas tree with all the ornaments that I love.

My usual activities are limited this year, and food just doesn't taste good, so I'm feeling a little ripped off. Danielle and her friend Austin have offered to put up the tree with Gene's help sometime soon, and I'm going to have to let go of some of the usual details. Gene tells me not to worry, because we are going to have one fantastic holiday season next year. He will take me wherever I want to go, and we will drag the kids with us. Doesn't get any better than that!

So I'm left with just one thing to do: rub it in that all my Christmas shopping is done and all my presents are wrapped!

Things People Don't Tell You

Monday, November 26: There are a number of things that no one tells you about when you are diagnosed with cancer. Top of the list is just how many doctor's appointments you will have. You feel like a hamster on one of those wheels running from appointment to appointment and getting closer to your goal—which is "Get this cancer out of me!"

I managed to skip a few steps because either I whined, people felt sorry for me, or I happen to know the system and I'm good at getting out of things. Take your pick. I wouldn't recommend anyone try this method. You must remember that I have a surgeon at my side at all times preventing me from doing something stupid. So I skipped the first step after finding a lump, which is to go to your primary care doctor. I happen to like my primary care doctor, but I like Gene better! I had Gene check the lump, and it was still there, so I scheduled a mammogram. I also got the routine detailed mammogram and sono in one appointment versus three. After that was the biopsy, which I did in one session rather than breaking it into two. Add oncology and surgeon's appointments, preop at hospital, doctor visits, EKG, and blood work, and this was all in a two-week period. Many people do it in less time than that. As a newly diagnosed cancer patient, you are literally in your car jumping from one appointment to another. As I told my children, "I have shown my chest to more people in two weeks than I have in over fifty years!" They only somewhat appreciate my humor.

The next thing people don't tell you about is the inability to sleep. I find myself with achy feet because I tiptoe around the house to keep from waking Gene and Dolly Dog. Dolly sighs a lot when I get up in the night. And some nights, she refuses to get up with me. I can't blame her. No sense in all of us being sleep deprived. Besides, Dolly and Gene have real jobs during the day, Gene as a surgeon and Dolly as a guard dog and companion extraordinaire.

One thing I didn't expect was that so many people would give me things. Seriously, a less respectful person could take advantage of this. I have been given so many gifts in the past month that it is mind-boggling. I have a collection in my office that I will repurpose someday. My new favorite (after the Dammit Doll, who gets a workout) is Pinkalicious, who was sent to me by a friend with whom I used to do motivational presentations on "Turning Lemons to Lemonade." Pinkalicious is going to be my chemo fairy, and I'm tying her to my chemo pole on Wednesday. I take her with my pink bubble gum to make sure everyone has a bubblicious day!

The Dammit Doll

Tuesday, November 27: My most humble and sincere apologies (is that overdoing it?) for not sharing my new friend with you sooner. Shortly after my diagnosis, my friend Debbie sent a Dammit Doll to me when I mentioned that I had some anger issues regarding my diagnosis. On the back of the doll, the tag reads:

Dammit Doll®
Whenever things don't go so well,
and you want to hit the wall and yell,
here's a little dammit doll,
that you can't do without.
Just grasp it firmly by the legs
and find a place to slam it.
And as you whack the stuffing out
yell "Dammit! Dammit! Dammit!"
www.dammitdolls.com

I find myself playing with the silly thing, and it always makes me smile. Too bad I'm not mad anymore!

Chemo Day

Wednesday, November 28: Today is chemo day number two, and I feel really, really good. Better than I have since surgery. So I really, really don't want to go to chemo. I hate this. Gene is leaving town this morning, and Tess is staying with me. I can't decide if I should put my game face on and waltz in there or if I should make her drag me kicking and screaming. I keep having these images of having a panic attack while they are doing a direct push of chemo meds and ending up with the nurse (connected to my port) and me wrestling on the floor. At least that vision amuses me.

I tolerated the first chemo session very well. As predicted by my physician, I felt fine for a couple of days, and then fatigue and nausea set in. Fortunately, the worst of it occurred over a weekend, and Gene was home to take care of me. My nausea was mostly controlled by medication, and I slept a lot. As I told my doctor, we can put that one in the win column.

Today is the second infusion and halfway point of phase one. I'm taking my chemo fairy and a large package of pink bubble gum with me. Oh, and don't forget that I'm taking Tess. We always find a way to have fun.

Making Chemo Fun!

Thursday, November 29: Tess was assigned to be my chemo buddy du jour, and we made the best of it. As we drove to chemo, we got stuck in a huge traffic jam coming off the interstate. We dodged, we weaved, and I shamelessly cut in front of other people. Tess waved out the window and said, "We're sorry, but my friend has cancer, and we don't want to delay her treatment." It was shocking, I tell you. We managed to squeak into chemo just in time despite the traffic. And then we began our entertainment.

I took with me my new "chemo fairy" and a large package of pink bubble gum. I assigned Tess the job of handing each person who came into our room a piece of bubble gum and wishing them a bubblicious day. It was too funny. Each person left with a big smile. I'm pretty sure we met people who didn't even have a place on my care team but wanted a piece of bubble gum. But who cares. I will take the smiles any way that I can get them.

We finished the day by tossing a few eggs at the forest. Tess agreed that there was something therapeutic about throwing eggs at trees.

Chemo Number Two Update

Saturday, December 1: Chemo number two went well, but it wiped me out. I came home and was supposed to spend some quiet time with friends, but I just wasn't up to it. Tess and Danielle encouraged me to at least eat the noodles out of my cup of soup. Then I headed for a three-hour nap. When I woke up, I did not recognize where I was or even who Tess was. I felt better, but I was back in bed by ten. So chemo days are exhausting.

I am required to go to the local hospital within twenty-four hours of chemo for an immune booster shot, and the next several days involve decreased energy and increased nausea. My roller coaster of side effects is a little different from the timeline the doctor predicted. I start feeling fatigue and nausea on day three, and it takes several days before I can function. The doctor has added a second nausea medication to help reduce the nausea, but the side effect is that I sleep all the time. I'm feeling better this morning, so hopefully today will bring a bit more energy.

Let Sleeping Dogs Lie

Sunday, December 2: I think of all the years my husband has rolled out of bed when he was called into the hospital during the night and taken care not to wake me. In the early years, every time the phone rang, I would wake up and have trouble going back to sleep. Then, as night-time phone calls became the norm in our house, I would just roll over and ignore the fact that he was dressing and leaving at one, two, or even four in the morning. Years later, I never even heard him get up.

Now I'm the nocturnal one. Steroids used to prevent complications from chemo keep me up at night. I find myself trying to perfect the "roll out of bed" without disturbing the covers. Some mornings, I even make a pretend me with the pillows to try to fool Gene. The problem is Dolly Dog. She has taken up residence next to my side of the bed to ensure I can't get up without stepping over her. And she has this new deer-antler treat, which she leaves just about anywhere. I squint, I scout, and I scan, but I manage to step on the pointy end frequently.

Finding quiet activities to occupy my mind at two to four in the morning has proven futile. Mostly I write blog entries. The clicking of the keyboard must drive Gene nuts, not to mention the light in the office. I tried the headlight/flashlight version, but it gave me a headache. So now I just try to shut the door to the bedroom while I'm roaming. But Dolly refuses to be shut in. Instead, she camps out near the office until the typing annoys her, and then with a sigh, she moves to the hall. She sighs a lot now.

Reading seems to be out of the question for now due to blurred vision—a chemo side effect that will go away in time. I find this extremely annoying since so many people have sent me great books to read and I'm an avid reader. So my only other activity is to bug my friends with early morning e-mails.

The Chemo Schedule

Wednesday, December 5: I get a lot of e-mails from people wanting to know how chemo is going. Well, that depends on the day. My chemo is currently scheduled every other Wednesday. When I get home from chemo, I'm exhausted, and eating seems to be too much effort. There is a touch of nausea, and all I want to do is lie down and take a rest. Thursday requires a trip to the hospital to get my immune-boosting shot, but otherwise, I feel just a touch of nausea. And then Friday hits. I get tired and nauseated. And by Saturday through Monday, I can barely lift my arms or stay awake, and the nausea seems to come and go. But the biggest issue is fatigue and the inability to get anything done.

I'm a person who likes to be doing several things at once, and I love a list of to-do items that I can mark off as I accomplish them. So the frustration level by Sunday/Monday is quite high. I called my mom yesterday and cried and told her it was too hard. Even holding the phone up to talk was too hard. I found myself leaning on the arm of the chair with my cell phone tucked on my shoulder. But then by noon on Tuesday, I was feeling a bit better. I actually wrapped two late-arriving presents. To be fair, they don't have bows, but the darn packages are wrapped, and I put that in the win column.

Today, Wednesday, a week after chemo, I feel like I'm going to live again. My appetite will return, but the mouth sores are going to be a problem. I'm even thinking of going out to dinner on Saturday night. The best part of chemo is that you can eat anything you want without feeling guilty. I'm down nearly thirty pounds so far. I have tossed out all the fat-free stuff, and I'm purchasing the full-fledged calorie-loaded pudding cups. Woo-hoo! But I still like sugar-free Jell-O. I like how it wiggles in my mouth! Yesterday I lived on popsicles. Today I plan to expand to some sort of real food.

The rest of the week leading back into chemo will get better and better until I charge into the Hall Perrine Cancer Center and tell them I'm ready to take over the world…and we start all over again.

Losing Hair Hurts and Other Things They Don't Tell You!

Wednesday, December 5: Just when you think you have suffered enough, chemo adds another insult. It turns out that losing your hair hurts. Actually hurts. I read up on it, and it seems that the hair follicles are the root (get it?) cause. I have read up on remedies, and here are my favorites:

- Use a lint roller—Seriously, this is like using a lint roller to pick up cat hair. Two swipes and it is full. But my short stubble does sort of resemble Wooly Willy, the magnetic pencil–metal shavings toy that you use to draw hair and a beard on the little face of the man. Except my shavings are coming off, not going on the head.
- Use duct tape—Ouch! You try it and get back to me.
- Use regular tape—This works to a point. I can pull large clumps of stubble off, but it still is mildly annoying.
- Wait it out—Sure, like I'm good at that!
- Rub mineral oil on it and massage—And then what? Spend the rest of the day leaving oil stains on the furniture and car headrest?

- Hot showers—This one I came up with on my own and feels the best. I don't know if it speeds up the dropping process, but at least for a few minutes, my scalp doesn't hurt.

Courage

Thursday, December 6: I keep hearing the words "courage" and "bravery" associated with me and find that ironic because I actually feel selfish. I'm not brave in this battle. I'm fighting for my life. Bravery is when you sacrifice for others. Our soldiers are brave. Our firefighters are brave. Our police are brave. I, on the other hand, just don't plan to die. I have things I want to do. So my only choice is in how I plan to face this battle.

I would like to say that I considered curling up in a ball and letting this all wash over me, but that isn't my nature. I'm more like a bull terrier with a chew toy—pulling and tugging and trying to manage the situation. I may not have the grace and elegance of Robin Roberts as she faces her battle, but I do have humor on my side. I have always looked at the world in a quirky way, and things that shouldn't, make me laugh. And usually when I'm laughing at inappropriate times, my friend Tess is at my side, and we are in stitches.

I don't have a bucket list, but I have started a small list of unfinished things I plan to do once chemo is over:

- Be on the *Ellen DeGeneres Show* and shamelessly plug my blog
- Get an e-mail from Robin Roberts saying I made her laugh
- Travel to Australia and New Zealand with Gene to celebrate our thirtieth anniversary (late)
- Write a book and dedicate it to my dad
- Put up the best Christmas tree ever next year (I have decided to go without a tree this year)
- Hug my children and thank my husband every chance I get

So call me strong. Call me determined. And please, oh please, call me funny. But don't call me brave.

I'm Done with That

Saturday, December 8: This is my notice to all worthwhile health-related causes that I will not be buying your logo wear or products from now on. When I pulled out my calendar at chemo the other day, my daughter looked at it, then at me, and said, "Do you realize that you have a breast cancer awareness calendar for 2012?" Oh yes, I realize it. Not only that, I already had a pink Iowa Hawkeye breast cancer ball cap and other related logo wear.

I'm not one that takes things as signs, but I'm telling you, from now on, I will *not* be buying anything that promotes awareness for lung cancer, heart disease, hangnail prevention, or typhoid. Just in case. No sir, you can keep your logo wear and products. I just ordered a nice, boring black calendar for next year!

Changing Expectations

Monday, December 10: Gene and I talked last night about how facing a year of chemo at this point can be daunting. My third session is quickly approaching, and I dread it. I had such a great weekend with our son and his girlfriend. We baked, we talked, we did things for other people, and we even went out to dinner. I felt almost normal again. But at the end of the weekend, we found ourselves planning for the upcoming chemo. Bummer.

That's when I told Gene that I simply could not focus on a year of this stuff but that breaking it into segments helped. He agreed and made some suggestions for focusing on the good days and what I can do on those days. Right now, I have about five bad days out of a fourteen-day cycle. These are days when I can't get much—or sometimes anything—done. So what *can* I do on the good days? Most people don't get the luxury of knowing when they are going to feel good and when they will feel bad, so this is an opportunity.

So today I'm taking a walk outside or getting on the recumbent bike for some exercise. I'm going to read some more of my book. (My eyesight is better at the end of the chemo two-week cycle than right after chemo.) I'm going to learn some new tricks in Photoshop—maybe put a bear into a photo of my front yard or make a tree disappear. Read up on bald-scalp care. Drop food off for the family we adopted for the holidays. Cook up a big pot of soup and freeze half of it. Make peanut brittle. And sing some Christmas carols. Take that, cancer!

Passing Time

Thursday, December 13: Chemo Day was fun and distracting. For some reason, it was quiet up there, and we started with the place to ourselves. I announced our arrival with a cheery "Here comes trouble!" Danielle and I tried out a new room and promptly sat the chemo fairy on the IV pole and got situated. It is starting to feel a little less surreal when we get there, but I hope to never get used to the routine. I tried to convince the doctor that a recumbent bike would be a good addition to the chemo area. Patients could take turns riding for five minutes. I worry that I will lose my mind when I have to start going there weekly.

My friend Karen came from Des Moines replete with artist supplies and informed Danielle and I that we would be doing an art project with our time. Karen is under the misconception that we all have hidden art talent inside of us. I have tried to explain to her on numerous occasions that this just might not be true. But the proof is in the pudding, as they say, and she was about to find a good dose of reality.

Karen hands Danielle and I each a white board and tells us to fill the page.

"With what?" I ask.

"Anything," Karen says. I look at her blankly. Danielle looks at the page. Karen says, "Let me start."

Oh sure. This is going to go well. Karen draws a series of lines and shapes that look quite nice. I grab my marker and draw a small squiggle. Not so bad. I add a Christmas tree, a Christmas yucca, an outline of my hand, and a coffee cup for the fun of it. Periodically, Karen flips my board sideways or upside down. I look at her board, and she has covered the white background, and it looks cool. Danielle has amazed me with a series of textures and patterns that look very artistic. My page looks like a coloring book drawn by a preschooler. But I get a compliment on my coffee-cup outline.

Then Karen gives us a paintbrush and tells us to paint shapes on top of our background. "Don't worry about smearing." Who is she kidding? I always worry about smearing. And I want a ruler! Karen's and Danielle's pieces are starting to look amazingly like art. Mine is a runny mess. Thank God it is lunchtime. Over lunch, Karen starts rethinking the project and says that maybe we should finish it next time. I'm laughing. I know defeat when I hear it. But it did make the time pass quickly! Karen might be able to pull this art project off with schoolchildren, but I am hopeless.

I'm Done with Cancer

Wednesday, December 19: Occasionally, people say they are sorry that I have cancer, and I stop for a second. I want to correct them and say, "No, I *had* cancer. Now I have chemo." But it would take too long to explain, so I let it go. The way Gene explains it to me is that the surgery removed the cancer, and for most patients, that should take care of things. But in a small percentage of patients, the cancer comes back. Unfortunately, the doctors don't know which patients will get a recurrence and which will be cured. Therefore, there is a chemo protocol that patients go through, depending on their type of breast cancer. I just drew some bad cards and have to go through a long series of chemo. So I'm so done with cancer. I have chemo.

Each chemo is a bit more difficult than the previous one. There seems to be a cumulative effect. I'm coming out of the bad days of chemo number three. Instead of four bad days like I had with the first and second infusion,

I had five-and-a-half bad days. But I'm on the uphill side and think I might actually accomplish a few things this week. I plan to help build a website but promise to leave the text editing to my son, just in case. I went to lunch with friends on both Monday and Tuesday. Both resulted in my having to come home and melt on the couch to recover, but it was so nice to have a normal lunch with girlfriends.

My doctor assures me that phase two of chemo is so much better and easier to tolerate than phase one. So I will tough it out and laugh my way through one more series and kiss phase one good-bye.

The Boredom Factor

Saturday, December 22: Thursday was an eventful day around our house. Eastern Iowa was hit with a full blizzard and a foot of snow. Our power went off at four in the morning, which launched us out of bed to get the fireplaces going. No dummies here. With over forty-eight hours' notice of the storm, we had stocked the basement and garage with plenty of firewood. So we at least had heat. And candles and lanterns are never a problem for two overly prepared people like Gene and me. Unfortunately, we didn't count on my boredom factor. After a couple of hours of sitting in the dark talking to each other, I got restless and started looking for something to do. My main focus was coffee.

The fireplace didn't have sufficient coals to boil a teakettle yet, so I had to improvise. I found a candle with three wicks and got to thinking. If caterers use small votive candles to heat chafing dishes, why couldn't a three-wick candle boil water? So I set up a stand using a small pot resting on a metal cooling rack (note the irony?) and propped it up over the candle. I can tell you that the water did eventually boil after one hour and fifteen minutes (and shortly after the actual power came on). Gene simply sat shaking his head and reminded himself that he was buying me an Etch a Sketch for Christmas.

Since the water was taking so long to boil, I decided to go the traditional method and use the coffeepot once the power came on. I sipped, I savored, and I enjoyed my first cup of coffee and the central heat as it warmed the house. I plugged every electronic device I owned into their chargers just in case the power was short lived. And I now had daylight to work with.

As I went in to enjoy a second cup of coffee and check the water-boiling progress, I smelled smoke. "Help! The coffeepot is on fire," I yelled to Gene, who came charging into the kitchen. (Please note that I'm talking about the real coffeepot. I did *not* set the house on fire with a candle and my improvised coffee device.) I pulled the plug, though this seemed a bit risky to me. Gene grabbed the boiling coffee carafe and then said, "Open the door." Out went the coffee maker, and we stood breathing deeply and looking at each other. And it was only quarter past eight. I no longer needed coffee to get my juices flowing. I was wide awake and ready for anything.

The remainder of the day was spent watching horizontal snow blow by, lighting candles as the power went out, stoking the fireplace, reading, and watching DVDs on my laptop. We ended up with twelve inches of snow and took the liberty of not removing it. With high winds, it was a waste of time anyway. It could wait until Friday morning.

The Last of Phase One

Thursday, December 26: It is the morning after Christmas and the day of my final chemo session in phase one, and I find myself not wanting to go in the worst way. I sit here at four in the morning and think of places to hide. I have had such a nice visit from the kids and felt really well for Christmas. It seems a shame to mess that up with chemo. It would be hard to describe the roller coaster of this first phase of chemo. Since I'm on dose-dense chemo, meaning my sessions are every two weeks rather than every three weeks, the breaks just don't seem long enough. I find it more difficult each time to walk in on one of my few good days and let them start treatment all over again. But today I remain focused on the fact that it is the last of the difficult chemo sessions, and I get to move on to something else in two weeks.

I'm taking all three of my children and Sam, my future daughter-in-law, with me to chemo today, and I have mixed emotions. The mom in me wants to protect them and hide this part of treatment from them. But I know they are adults, and I treasure their company. So off to chemo we will go. They are bringing card games to entertain me with, so I know the time will pass quickly. I wonder who will have to be bubblicious today and pass out the bubble gum. Shall we make sweet Sam do it? She always has a smile on her face, so that doesn't seem very challenging. Shall we make Steven be bubblicious? I suspect he would be a good sport, but it would be a toss-up as to whether him or Nick would be more bugged by being the center of attention. Danielle has already had a turn. Quite frankly, I make someone do this just because I can. It amuses me. Maybe I will take pity on them and just put the bubble gum on the counter.

So imagine me with my chin thrust forward and determination in my eye as I march into chemo today. Take that, cancer! You have not defeated me yet.

I Survived Phase One!

Friday, January 4, 2013: The last chemo session of phase one was hard to recover from. It has taken me eight days to work up the energy to write. I sort of feel like Punxsutawney Phil, the groundhog, coming out of my tunnel and looking for my shadow. Is it spring yet? It took a full week before I was feeling human again. The nausea is mostly controlled by medication, but the antinausea medication puts me to sleep about half an hour after I take it. So I went from sleeping in the chair, to the sofa, to the chair, to the bed, and so forth for the last week. But yesterday, I was drug-free. And what did I do with myself?

I decided to start exercising again. You should know by now that I don't do anything in moderation. Full steam ahead is my theory. I decided to join the walking group at the local skate arena. Having never been there before, I imagined an ice-skating rink that you walk around. So I bundled up and grabbed my walking shoes. Imagine my surprise when I walked into a nice, climate-controlled roller rink. At least they don't require skates! I took off several layers of clothing and joined the walkers going in circles. My initial goal was to walk about fifteen minutes and take my time. But the old ladies, and I mean people in their eighties, were passing me, and it ticked me off.

I'm nothing if not competitive, and there was no way I was letting someone who looked like they were recovering from a hip transplant pass me. The problem was, they just kept going, and I was running out of steam! There was a time when I could walk at a good four-miles-per-hour clip and do a mile in fifteen minutes. My new goal was to not embarrass myself by arriving after and leaving before the geriatric crowd. Granted, there weren't any other chemo-induced bald people there who I could identify. But pride is pride.

After thirty minutes, I was exhausted and had to call it quits. I was relieved to see a few other people leaving. I staggered out after them. A friend invited me for coffee, but I declined and went home to lick my wounds in private. Wobbly knees and an achy hip tell me that my first goal of fifteen minutes may have been the rational goal. But what the heck. If it doesn't kill you...

CHAPTER 4
CHEMOTHERAPY PHASE TWO

Starting Chemo Phase Two

Thursday, January 10, 2013: Now that I'm finished with phase one of chemo, it is time to start phase two. My doctor assures me that phase two will be easier to tolerate than phase one, and I admit that I am breathing a sigh of relief to be done with the first phase. While there were only four infusions in phase one, the cumulative effect made each infusion more difficult than the previous one. Phase two consists of weekly infusions for twelve weeks. Once again, my doctor has given me a list of possible side effects in phase two:

- Fatigue
- Hair loss (my hair is already gone, so this one doesn't worry me)
- Nausea/vomiting (but less than in phase one)
- Increased risk of infection
- Anemia
- Increased risk of bleeding
- Heart dysfunction
- Skin/nail changes
- Numbness/tingling in hands/feet
- Body aches
- Allergic reaction

Because of the risk of allergic reaction, I am asked to bring a driver with me for the first two visits. My sister has volunteered to fly in from Texas and go with me to my first appointment. We don't get nearly enough time together, so this will be fun. My husband also chose to take the day off in case I have an allergic reaction. I feel safer knowing he will be there.

When I walk into the infusion area, the nurses note that this is my first infusion of Taxol, and they mark my room with a big sign that says "#1." As the nurses start my IV and bring in my meds, each one remarks that they will be watching me closely today. I'm starting to get nervous.

Phase two infusions start with premeds to help me tolerate the chemo. I am given medicine for nausea and heartburn and a couple medicines to prevent allergic reactions. I count five bags of premeds and two bags of chemo marked as hazardous materials. One of the primary premeds is Benadryl, which makes me very groggy. Once all the premeds have been administered, it is time for the chemo medication. Since this chemo has a history of allergic reactions in patients, a nurse is assigned to sit with me for the first fifteen minutes. She reads me a list of possible signs of allergic reaction and tells me to tell her immediately if I feel even the least bit funny. Then she watches me.

At this point, my heart is beating quickly, and I'm feeling like a fish in a fishbowl. The nurse is looking at me, my husband is looking at me, and my sister is looking at me. I have no urge to joke with them, but I would like them to quit staring at me. Every few minutes the nurse asks if I'm feeling okay. Seriously, you are starting to freak me out! I'm really, really sleepy, but I'm afraid if I go to sleep, someone will hit me with the heart paddles to wake me.

After the first ten to fifteen minutes, the nurse tells me I'm doing well and leaves the room. Nap time! I crank up my seat heater and vibrator, and off to sleep I go. Gene rests his eyes as he sits in the corner. My sister takes this time to go exploring. She has inherited the same trait I have in that she gets bored easily. When I wake up, my sister tells me there is a video loan program on the first floor where I can borrow videos to watch during chemo. And she says the gift store and wig store have some really cute items. She has seen more of this building than I have!

Six hours after walking in the door, we are finally finished. We are all hungry and exhausted, so we go to a restaurant to get lunch/dinner. I'm so tired that I just stare at my food and watch Gene and Danielle eat. But I survived the first of twelve infusions in phase two.

Breasts Come in Hatboxes

Saturday, January 5: I decided it was time to go get fitted for a prosthetic breast. I have been using the bra inserts that the hospital gave me, which are made of quilt batting and a piece of Velcro that slip into your camisole or bra. The problem with the inserts is that they don't stay in place but tend to wander to your shoulder or under your armpit when you sit down. My daughter has a sign she gives me when we are in public that means, "Mom, your breast is on your shoulder." There have been occasions when I have been tempted to fake an Alzheimer's moment and ask loudly, "What? My breast has gone AWOL?"

So anyway, I arrive at the prosthetic store and take a deep breath and walk in. The nice lady asks how she can help me. I kid you not. I'm so tempted to say, "I'd like a breast to go." But I behave myself and tell them that I'm there for a breast prosthetic. I provide my insurance and prescription, and they show me to a large fitting room. I find it funny that you have to have a prescription to buy a breast prosthetic. Who other than a mastectomy patient would want one?

I'm told to remove my shirt. Here we go again: yet another in a series of strangers who gets to look at my chest. Someone once told me that when you have cancer, the indignities never end. I'm starting to get their point.

I'm not sure what to expect at this point, but I suspect there will be a lot of measuring and maybe a mold of my other breast. Not so much. It turns out they do have takeout! The lady checks to make sure my incision has healed sufficiently to wear a prosthetic and asks my bra size. She hands me a robe and leaves. I don't know whether to be disappointed that I don't have "special" breasts or to be grateful that I might actually be able to leave looking normal. I sit down to wait.

We all know by now that waiting isn't my strength. As I look around, I notice a breast sitting in a cup next to me. I glance at the door. I glance back at the breast. Yep, I'm picking it up. (You know you would too!) It feels amazingly lifelike. And I'm intrigued by the little massage bubbles on the back side. They look remarkably like the air pockets in my shoe inserts. Cool! I hold the breast up next to my chest and think that this might work better than I thought. I look around to see what other toys they have left within my reach and find...nipple expanders. An eyebrow goes up. That sounds painful. The door opens before I can explore further.

The nice lady walks in with an assortment of bras and a hatbox. I'm intrigued. My new breast comes in a pink hatbox? How cute is that? The lady opens the box, and the prosthetic looks huge. I guess I hadn't thought about it, but it wasn't just the breast they removed but rather all the tissue on the chest wall and under my arm. She inserts the prosthetic in a special pocket in the bra and helps me try it on. I say "helps" because this thing is made of ballistics gel and weighs quite a bit. We walk to the mirror, and she asks what I think. Now that is a dangerous question.

My standards are pretty low at this point. For two months I have been chasing quilt batting around my shoulder and chest or simply been going lopsided. I tell her that I think the breast is in the right general area and I'm happy. Not so fast. These people are professionals, and they aren't going to let me leave without perfection. She calls in an assistant. Back to showing my chest to strangers. They decide I need a different bra and leave. Fine by me. More time to explore.

Now there are two ladies shoving ballistics gel into a bra and asking me to try it on. They seem happier. They take a satin robe, put it on me backward, and pull it tight against my chest, and we all stare at my bustline in the mirror. I manage to keep my mouth shut. They tell me they want to make sure I don't "muffin-top" out. Sounds good. Mouth shut, but I'm dying to entertain them. They keep commenting on how good my attitude is, and I want to tell them they haven't even seen my attitude yet. So I start joking around with them, and it turns out they have pretty good senses of humor.

We talk about what insurance will cover. A breast prosthetic runs $425 regardless of size. They are good to help with insurance. They tell me that my insurance will also cover a wet prosthetic for swimming. Oh boy, uncharted territory. I decide to hold off. After all, it is minus-two degrees outside and a bit soon to think about swimming. And why have all the fun in one day? My sister and I could really tear the place up with laughter over "wet prosthetics."

So it turns out that my new breast is supposed to sleep facedown in its hatbox overnight and be washed after wearing each day. But it is a massage form, so I get a free massage every day, and the gel is supposed to make it cooler in the summer. I will have to let you know.

My friend Teri asked me if the hatbox was more top hat or sombrero shaped, so I sent her a photo and reserved comment!

The Sister

Monday, January 14: My sister is visiting from Texas, and we are having a blast. Long conversations, visits to our favorite haunts, and lots of laughs have filled our days. It has been a nice distraction from chemo.

While we were out shopping today, I decided to stop and fill my van up with fuel. I pulled up to the pump and jumped out to fill the tank. Tammy picked up her cell phone to check messages while she was waiting. She was texting away when she suddenly felt someone staring at her. She looked up, and the man at the pump in front of us was glaring at her. She felt that was odd but decided to ignore him. He glared harder. She glanced up and was wondering what his problem was, when he glanced at me, then back at her. She looked over her shoulder and saw her bald sister standing out in the cold January weather filling the car while she was casually texting away. The man continued to glare at her.

About this time, I open the door to drop my credit card in my purse. Tammy points out that the man is glaring at her and asks if I could I hurry up, and I start laughing. When I get in the car, he continues to give her the evil eye, and I can't stop laughing. He assumes I need help, and Tammy knows that I wouldn't let her put gas in my car unless I was in two leg casts. Having cancer isn't a disability; it is just a big, darn inconvenience at times. I turn to her and ask, "Do you want me to tell him you don't have legs?" We continue to laugh as we drive off.

We come home and decide it would be a good day to blow some pumpkins up. We toss in a red poinsettia and a spaghetti squash just for the fun of it. Blowing things up continues to be therapeutic.

The Red Balloon

Friday, January 18: Those of you who know me know that I love symbolism and a good theme. While I have enjoyed blowing things up after each chemo round, I find the temperatures in the single digits take some of the fun out of it. So I have had to come up with something symbolic to do after each treatment in phase two. I decided to take my friend Marion's suggestion and channel my inner Pooh: "So remember Winnie the Pooh and his red balloon floating up and away…when your cares are too heavy, just tie them up in that balloon and watch it going up, up, and away!" wrote Marion.

I plan to release one red balloon every week for the next twelve weeks when I get home from chemo to represent one more step toward remission. Then, after my last session in phase two, I plan to release an entire bouquet of red balloons and laugh and clap as they go up, up, and away.

When your cares are too heavy, tie them up in a balloon and watch it going up, up, and away.

Week Three

Saturday, January 26: My outdoor thermometer read minus-zero degrees today, and I spent some time trying to decide how zero could be a negative number. How much warmer would it have to be to read plus-zero? Ultimately, I decided that it was too cold for me to release balloon number three, and I asked Gene to do it for me. I tried to toss in a pitiful cough to go along with it, but he wasn't buying it. He was a good sport and took the balloon out into the wind, and we watched it sail away. Say good-bye to week three of chemo.

I could not imagine going through chemo without the wonderful friends and family who are helping me. Dog sitters, chemo sitters, food preparers, letter writers, bloggers, drivers, medicine getters, prayers, and balloon tossers. So many people offering support in so many ways. I truly appreciate all of their support.

The Bell

Tuesday, January 29: There is a bell that hangs just inside the doorway of the chemotherapy floor, and I look at it with longing each time I pass it. It looks a lot like a ship's bell, with a chord hanging down just waiting to be rung. But this isn't an ordinary bell. It is a symbol of completion. Each chemo patient gets to ring the bell on his or her final day of chemotherapy.

When the bell is rung, everyone stops what they are doing and claps. The staff has huge smiles on their faces as they celebrate with the patient the end of a journey and the start of a new journey. A couple of weeks ago, I heard the bell ring, and I felt a moment of sadness that it wasn't my turn. Then I immediately started to clap, and a big smile came across my face. The bell represents hope. I cannot wait to ring the bell.

Return to Normalcy

Saturday, February 2: I saw an interview with Robin Roberts yesterday in which she mentioned that the one thing she craved was the return to normalcy, and I thought, "That's it! That is what I want." I want a day where chemotherapy never enters my mind. A day where I don't worry that I will come into contact with someone who has the flu. A day where I'm not trying to figure out how to drink three-fourths of a gallon of fluids to flush my liver and kidneys. A day where on a whim I can buy an airline ticket to Texas to visit my family.

But on the other hand, I have to admit that I'm feeling pretty good in this phase of chemo. I don't feel sick or particularly tired. I go through most days without a nap, and I'm working again on the days when my vision isn't blurred. So I really don't have anything to complain about.

I wonder how long it will be after chemo ends before I feel like things return to normal. When will I not worry about cancer? Just for the record, I feel like my cancer is gone. I continue through the treatments because I want to ensure it never comes back. Week four of twelve is done with, and I have launched my red balloon into my neighbor's woods! I wonder how many balloons they will find next spring.

Sleeping like the Dead

Monday, February 4: Thursday was a long day at chemo. The day started with difficulty in getting my port to cooperate. My port is located in my chest, and that is where the nurses insert the IV medicines. Jody, my nurse extraordinaire, showed a lot of patience and persistence in trying to get my port to cooperate. After a couple of hours, we decided to start a standard

IV and get the show on the road.

Chemotherapy can involve multiple medicines and IV bags as well as premedications to help prevent side effects. One of the premeds that I take is a hefty dose of IV Benadryl. Unfortunately, a small dose of Benadryl knocks me out on a normal day. And if you give me a large dose while I am seated in a chair with seat warmers and a vibrator, I sleep like the dead. Literally.

So on Thursday, the doctor comes in to speak with me and check my port. She sees that I am sleeping and calls my name. Nothing. I don't move. She gently shakes my arm and calls my name again. Nope. I'm not waking up. The nurse shakes my arm and calls my name. I sleep on. Now everyone is looking a little concerned, and the doctor lifts her stethoscope. At this point, my sweet daughter, Danielle, grabs my arm and shouts, "Mom!" I sit straight up. Nothing like the sound of your child bellowing your name to get a mom up and running! I look around at the room full of people smiling at me and say, "Oh, hi." I have no idea that I have just scared them to death.

I'm thinking I should leave instructions in my will that someone should check me twice to make sure I'm really dead.

Entertainment

Tuesday, February 12: For those of you who know me well, you know that I'm truly happy when I'm doing two or three things at once. I'm not very good at sitting still or being idle for long periods of time. This was one of my biggest concerns about chemotherapy. When Dr. Nabi told me that my weekly chemo appointments would last about four hours, I wondered what I would do to entertain myself. I remember asking her in the early weeks if she would consider getting a stationary bike for the chemo floor. She smiled and said no but that I was welcome to walk around (with my IV pole). Now that I have been in chemo for a while, I see her point. Most of the people getting chemo actually look ill. Go figure. I, on the other hand, charge in there like I'm storming a bridge.

Like so often in my life, my friends have come to the rescue. Several of them take turns going to chemo with me and providing entertainment. Some have gotten very creative.

Last week, my friend Kassia came to the rescue with yarn and knitting needles and the claim that she was going to teach me to "knit poorly." I'm in! This sounds like there are fewer expectations of a useable product at the end. She told me that she bought very "forgivable" yarn, which also sounds like a good idea. Because I fell asleep after the infamous Benadryl, I only learned how to go one direction. When I got home and picked up the knitting, I realized I didn't know how to turn around and go the other direction. So I think I can knit something really long and skinny. I did e-mail her and ask for directions on how to turn around, and I think I may have accomplished it. But I suspect this scarf is getting narrower and narrower as I work along.

I have played card games with my kids, talked with friends, slept through daytime television, and worked on crossword puzzles. I posted a request for entertainment ideas to occupy me during chemo on my blog. I have seven sessions in phase two left to go.

Chocolate

Thursday, February 14: Because it is Valentine's Day, I thought I would talk about one of my biggest fears with chemo. Ever since I started chemotherapy, I have lost my love for chocolate. This is horrible and frightening to me. Chocolate just doesn't taste good, and I'm a bit upset by the whole thing. You have to understand that chocolate is a basic food group in my life. I allow myself one bite of chocolate a day. I can make a candy bar last an entire week, which makes my husband crazy. (He makes me crazy when he walks by my open candy bar and eats it, claiming he assumed I didn't want it.) What if I never love chocolate again? Is life without chocolate even possible?

Iowa Winters

Monday, February 18: I hate winter in Iowa. It just seems so unreasonable that you have to wear a coat for six to seven months a year. I usually get stir-crazy in January, and Gene plans a trip to someplace where you don't have to wear a parka, gloves, a scarf, and a fur-lined hat just to go to the grocery store. I ask him to take me somewhere south of Oklahoma so I can walk outside and feel the wind on my face and in my hair. I practically kiss the ground when we land someplace warm.

This year, we have been limited in where we can travel due to risk of the flu or norovirus while flying. With a compromised immune system, I have been very careful about where I go. But we have managed to take two weekends to get away. The first one was to Illinois (marginally south of Iowa) to go wedding dress shopping with my future daughter-in-law and her mother. It was so exciting to get away and do something normal. I did tire easily, but it was well worth getting out of town for.

Then last weekend, Gene took me to Des Moines to have dinner with friends and visit some of our favorite haunts. When we checked into the hotel, the desk clerk asked us what brought us to Des Moines. Without blinking, I told him we were going south for the winter! He laughed and asked if we were from Minnesota. "No," I explained, "we live near Cedar

Rapids," and he laughed harder. Des Moines is exactly forty miles south and one hundred miles west of our house. So in my opinion, we went to the Southwest for a weekend.

Gene and I were supposed to be in Hawaii this month, and it is disappointing not to be able to go. I knew this chemo thing was going to put a major dent in my travel schedule, but you find your fun where you can. We had fun in Illinois and Des Moines, and Hawaii will be taking reservations for next year very soon. And a year from now, my hair will have grown back, I will be able to walk in the breeze with my face pointed toward the sky, and chemo will be a distant memory.

Chemo Cocktail

Friday, February 22: Each week, I receive a complicated mix of premeds and chemo meds. I watch as the IV bags arrive and the nurses sort them out. Some IVs last five minutes. Some last thirty minutes. The nurses keep them straight, checking and double-checking them, and I no longer worry about what they are hanging.

Last week, my nurse Jodie came in with my chemo meds and announced that she had my cocktail ready. I looked at her and said, "I normally like olives with my cocktail and straight up!" She laughed and said she did too. This week as my chemo meds arrived, Jodie walked in and said she had something for me. She pulled out a jar of olives, and we both laughed. I have the best nursing care on earth! We find fun wherever we can.

The Nurses

Monday, March 4: I have the best nursing care in the world. Each visit to chemotherapy, I have a team of about six or seven nurses who take care of me. I couldn't begin to name them all, but a few of them work with me each week. Molly is who I call if I have unusual or significant side effects. She knows I hate to call but has convinced me that it is important and can reduce serious complications. She also knows that I will never call at night or over the weekend unless I think I'm dying. Yet she encourages me to pick up the phone before that point and promises to point out to the doctor that I was a good girl and actually called before arriving at death's door.

Ashley takes my vitals every week and is the evil one who makes me step on the scale. I sigh and pray to the scale gods to be kind. She keeps up with my blog and laughs with me at some of my antics and observations.

Laurie is the first nurse I met when I started chemo. She is confident and fun. She asks if I'm going to cause trouble, to which I respond, "Of course." But she greets me with a smile anyway. She assures me that the nurses fight over who gets me for the week. I'm sure that is true, but I'm not sure if they are fighting because they want to get me or they don't want to get me for a patient. We celebrate when my port cooperates and commiserate when it doesn't.

Jody is the other nurse I get each week. She is persistent and determined to conquer my port. My sister calls her a "keeper" because she fought my port until she was able to get it to work. Others would have given up long before then. Jody always greets me with a smile and laughs when I'm sarcastic. She brings my cocktail of meds each week.

I have many more nurses who care for me weekly, as well as receptionists and schedulers. They all seem to like their jobs and work hard to call me by name. I like all my nurses, and they make me feel welcome, safe, and well cared for.

Labs

Friday, March 8: Each week, after I check into reception, my first stop is to get labs. There is a nice, big, sunny waiting room where everyone is waiting for their name to be called. Most people come with a friend or family member, and I entertain myself by deciding which person has cancer and is here for treatment and which one is the support team.

Sometimes it is easy: the patient is bald. I score only one point for getting these right. Sometimes I look for the one who is in a wheelchair or who looks ill. I get two points for getting these right because about a third of the time, this is the friend or chemo buddy. And my favorite guessing game is the healthy-looking couples. I credit myself five points for getting these right. One by one, the lab techs come out and call a name, and I decide how many points I get. It passes the time.

Since this waiting room seems rather quiet and solemn, I have decided to liven things up a bit. Now when a lab tech comes out to call a name, I throw my hands up and say, "Pick me, pick me!" This makes most people laugh. (I'm sure they are wondering what premeds I took that morning and if they can ask the doctor for some.) The lab techs laugh and shake their heads. This week, the lab tech stuck her head out and said, "Kathy L. Come on down!" and we both laughed.

Labs are labs, just like at any doctor's appointment. They draw the blood, put a cotton ball on it, and have you apply pressure for five minutes because chemo can make you clot slower. They apply a piece of tape to your arm, and you are on your way. Except this week something new happened.

As I am sitting there waiting for my blood to clot (sounds entertaining, doesn't it?), I hear a noise and look over to see a canister pop out of a vacuum tube like they have at the drive-through at the bank. My eyes get wide, and I cock my head. What could that be for? I ask one of the techs, and she tells me that if they have samples they can't process on this floor, they put them in the tube, which goes to the hospital. Now you have to realize, these samples have to travel three floors down and half a block down the street to reach the hospital. Cool!

I start to think about this and ask the tech, "Have you ever put something other than samples in there?"

She asks, "Like what?"

I ask if she has ever put Smarties (the candy) or pennies in there. Think of the noise it would make as it rattled down three floors, through the lobby, down the street, and into the hospital halls and lab! Can you just see yourself walking down a hospital corridor with this rattling going by?

The lab tech looked at me, smiled, and said, "I think that would be an OSHA violation." Too bad. I tell her that is why I can't work someplace that has rules and have to work from home.

The Promise

Sunday, March 10: A long time ago, during our second winter in Iowa, we had a late, heavy snowstorm in April on the day of the school carnival. I wasn't used to Iowa winters yet and was surprised when I got home with three children to find the driveway blocked by a three-foot snow furrow left by the snowplow. The snow was heavy and wet, and there was no way my van could cross it. I parked the van in the middle of the road and lifted the children over the drift, and we made our way to the house. They were too young to be of help removing snow, so I grabbed boots and a shovel and went to work digging out. Gene was on call at the hospital.

An hour later, I was standing in the driveway sobbing and cursing the great state of Iowa and my husband, who moved us here. Neighbors were calling the house to ask the kids if I was okay. When my husband called to check in later that evening, I threatened to leave him *and* make him keep the children if he didn't get me out of the snow soon. He quickly realized that I am greatly affected by SAD (seasonal affective disorder—or, as I like to think of it, snow again, dammit!)

Two things resulted from this incident. On Monday, a shiny, brand-spankin'-new self-propelled snowblower that was capable of throwing three feet of snow for miles arrived. This machine had features that my neighbors would envy for years. And second, Gene promised me that he would take me out of the great state of Iowa on a vacation every January or February to a location of my choosing—which was anywhere south of Oklahoma. He has kept that promise for the past nineteen years, and we always look forward to that trip and getting away from the snow. I find that this trip changes my attitude, and soon he, the kids, and the great state of Iowa aren't so bad after all.

Unfortunately, my chemo schedule has not allowed us to travel this winter, except for a couple of weekend trips to Des Moines and Champaign, Illinois, both marginally south. To add insult to injury, we had to cancel our February trip to Hawaii. I admit, I pouted.

All this leads to my dilemma. Tuesday is our thirtieth anniversary, and I want to do something fun to celebrate it. So I posted my dilemma on my blog, hoping Team Kathy could help come up with ideas that didn't require travel. As always, my team didn't disappoint me. I received multiple suggestions on how to bring Hawaii to me. But my favorite suggestion came from a friend who suggested we get in the car and go to the car wash. How creative!

Double Digits

Monday, March 18: Last week, the doctor and nurses greeted me with the news that I had entered double digits (like I hadn't been counting!). Thursday was my tenth chemo session in phase two. It was a big week for me because now I am close enough to see the end of phase two on the horizon. There are several more steps before I finish chemo. But we take our accomplishments where we can find them, and this milestone is noteworthy. Only two more sessions before I get to take a three-week break. Then I start radiation.

The side effects of the chemo are starting to get worse, as I feel tired more easily and mild nausea is a constant companion. But I'm still feeling better than I anticipated I would feel at this point. I think a winning attitude helps, as well as the support of family and friends. And Dolly Dog is always willing to take an afternoon nap with me.

This week was also Daffodil Day for the American Cancer Society. The local ACS was very sweet to provide every chemo patient with a dozen daffodils in their chemo room to take home. Two ladies from the society came by to make sure I knew what resources were available to me at the Hall Perrine Cancer Center. I'm not sure what they were expecting, but they got more than they bargained for when they entered my room. I had them laughing hard, and they seemed embarrassed to laugh at my cancer jokes. Jodie, my nurse, just shook her head at them and said, "She is bad." I figure that no one gets to feel sorry for me in my room. They have to laugh with me. The ladies left just shaking their heads.

When I got home, the bank ladies brought me a dozen daffodils as well, which I so much appreciated. The house is filled with these bright-yellow pops of spring and the promise that we might survive the winter. The cards that are included say that daffodils bring hope—hope of a cure, hope of remission, hope of survival. I share that hope. I told my husband I hoped I would be the last breast cancer patient. I could take this so much easier if I knew my journey saved others.

Gene and I walked to the top of the hill, where we released my tenth red balloon and watched it sail away. I think Winnie the Pooh was right: you can watch all your troubles sail away as that balloon lifts up, up, and away.

The Eleventh Balloon

Tuesday, March 26: Each week after chemo, I launch a red balloon into the air to signify the end of another infusion and being one step closer to remission. Most weeks, I'm so exhausted after chemo that I just come home and go to sleep and save the balloon for the weekend. I have amused myself by letting the balloons go on different parts of our hill and watching them fly away.

Over the weekend, I asked Gene to drive me over the Cedar River bridge so I could release the balloon from the car window. I thought it would be fun to see it fly over the river. So we loaded up and took the balloon for a ride. As we neared the bridge, Gene slowed down, and I rolled down the window and stuck the balloon out. The wind grabbed the balloon immediately, and I watched in the rearview mirror as it crossed over the bridge.

Just then, Gene says, "Uh-oh." When I ask what is uh-oh, he tells me that there is a police car with his lights on behind us. Ha-ha! He is so funny. Then I look in the rearview mirror and see that there really is a police car speeding toward us with its lights on. I'm holding my head, saying, "Oh no! Oh no!" over and over again, and wondering if I should pull the cancer card and take my hat off so my bald head shows. Gene tells me to relax because the sheriff isn't after us.

As the sheriff's car passes us, I ask, "What are the odds of getting caught at something like this?"

Gene glances at me and says, "With you in the car? Pretty good."

Thursday is my last weekly chemo infusion and the end of phase two. I get a three-week break to recover, and then I start daily radiation and chemo every three weeks. I plan to celebrate by releasing a dozen red balloons with some friends on Friday. I think we will stay on my own property and not get creative.

Ringing the Bell

Sunday, March 7: March 28 was my last weekly chemo in phase two, and my mom was here from Texas to celebrate with me. It was a fun day at chemo as everyone came in to congratulate me. The nurses try to make it as much of a celebration as possible by signing a certificate of completion and blowing bubbles at you as you get ready to leave. All the patients applaud and smile as you walk by. And then it is time to ring the bell. You should know that I had no intention of going quietly or being subtle when I rang the bell. I am glad to be done with weekly chemo, and I planned to show it!

When I got to the bell, I grasped hold of the chord and rang it for all I was worth. My ears were ringing, and my eyes were watering from the noise, but it was worth it to hear everyone laugh. Then I turned to the nurses and said, "I will see you on Monday," and they all laughed harder. (I have a research study appointment there on Monday.) When we walked through the reception area, everyone was looking up to see who had finished chemo, and they applauded as well. It is rather embarrassing to know I rang the bell so hard they could hear me half a building away! In fact, the first photos we shot are nothing but a blur of a crazy lady at the bell.

While I am not totally done with chemo, it was so nice to celebrate the end of the "hard stuff." Phase three is in two parts. I take a three-week break, and then I start daily radiation for six-and-a-half weeks. I will also have chemo every three weeks, but without most of the side effects that I have had with phases one and two. Stay tuned for the fun Gene has in store for me to celebrate the end of each week of radiation.

Celebrating the End of Phase Two of Chemo

Wednesday, April 3: One of the things that amuses me is that when temperatures in the spring reach forty degrees, people in Iowa start taking their coats off and talking about how nice the weather is. I suspect we are all just happy to have survived the long winter. On Friday, God granted us one of those beautiful spring days with calm winds and temperatures near fifty. It was a perfect day to celebrate the end of phase two of chemo with friends.

A bunch of girlfriends and my mom gathered with me to release a dozen red and pink balloons to signify the end of twelve chemo rounds in phase two. I also released one white balloon as a tribute to all breast cancer patients who have gone before me and helped define my treatment. Many women have volunteered for research studies (as have I) to help future patients with treatments. I wanted to pay tribute to them for making the road a bit easier for me and for improving my survival chances.

One of the best treats of the day was that I got to meet my cyber breast cancer mentors, Julie and Chris. They both took the day off and came out and helped launch the balloons. They have been so helpful and supportive of me through this process. I have truly enjoyed my nontraditional support group.

After releasing the balloons and having a champagne toast, we all went to lunch and chatted and laughed and had such a great time. I'm so glad my mom could be here for the last week to help me out and to visit. She says she feels better leaving this time because I am doing so well. Today was truly a day of celebration.

CHAPTER 5
RADIATION THERAPY

My New Tattoos

Thursday, April 11, 2013: I have my radiation simulation done today, and it was quite interesting—you might even call it life altering. The staff introduces themselves and shows me to a room where I am told to remove everything from the waist up. They provide me with a chic, soft pink cape that opens in the front. The best part is that the cape is made of fleece and is toasty warm. Finally, a place that has chic capes that keep you warm!

I do not know what to expect in my "simulation," but the word implies that they are going to show me how my radiation treatments are going to go. Well, not so much…

I am shown into the CT scan room and told to lie down on the comfy, hard metal table with my head resting near the open end of what looks like a science fiction machine that sucks your brains out. While I'm familiar with what CT scans do, the process still doesn't seem like a good idea to me. The doctor and staff come in and explain what they are going to do today. They will take some images and photos and then tattoo my skin with permanent marks so that they can radiate the exact position of my chest each time. I perk up. Tattoos?

My arms are positioned over my head, and the staff explain that the CT scan table will move in and out of the big circle CT scanner. I'm told that I should lie still but breathe normally and that the scan will take only about five minutes. Do these people know what kind of trouble I can get into in five minutes? Then they tell me that while they won't be in the room with me, they will be able to see and hear me the entire time. Well, that certainly limits what mischief I will get into!

The staff leaves, and the table moves in and out, finding the right position, then stops, and the test begins. This entertains me for about a minute, and then I'm bored and my mind wanders. I start looking closer at the CT scanner, wondering how it works, when I notice a label on the inside. My glasses are off, and the label is upside down. But I have nothing better to do, so I squint and decipher: "Do not stare directly into laser as it may cause permanent eye damage." What? This label is located right next to a red light! If I can read the label, I'm probably "staring directly into the laser." And shouldn't that label be facing the other direction? Breathing normally is out of the question.

The technician enters the room, and before I can ask about the laser label, I notice a digital camera in her hand. This can't be good. She tells me that she is going to take some photos for my file. My "file" sounds a lot like my "permanent record," and there is no way I want topless photos in my permanent record. She takes the photos, and I wonder if these photos will somehow surface if I ever run for political office. Or what if I ever have to testify before Congress, and they ask if I have ever had nude photos taken? I'm not liking this, but the tech quickly moves on to discussing tattoos, and she has my undivided attention again.

The tech tells me she is going to put three tattoos on me. I promptly ask for a butterfly and a flower, and for the third, I'm torn between a heart and Gene's initials. I'm told that all I'm getting is three dots so they can line me up properly for each radiation treatment. Bummer! And I don't even get to pick the color of the dots! Fifty-three years without a tattoo, and now they are taking all the fun out of it.

Let me tell you, the tattoos hurt. Not the kind of hurt where it brings tears to your eyes but enough that you wonder why anyone would willingly go in and get one. I get a dot in each side of my rib cage and one in the cleavage area. The tech tells me that there is a smear of ink in each area but that it will wash off. I'm told to go change back into my clothes.

Of course, the first thing I do in the changing room is look at my new tattoos in the mirror. The ink smears are distracting, so I wet a paper towel to wipe them away. The water doesn't take much of the ink away, but I notice the hand-sanitizing liquid and remember that alcohol removes ink. Now let me just say that I was intent on seeing my new tattoos and not thinking this through clearly. I wet the towel with sanitizer, wipe the tattoo area, and nearly fall to my knees as the alcohol hits the open wound. Have you ever tried to blow on your own rib cage? I'm prancing around the changing room trying to fan my tattoos and not cry.

I leave with my calendar of thirty-three radiation appointments and five other appointments and wonder what I did with my time before doctor's appointments. I'm heading to Target to buy some temporary rub-on tattoos to surprise Gene with. Do you think I should put Hello Kitty or Dora the

Explorer in my cleavage?

Spring Break—The Great Escape

Wednesday, April 17: I have three weeks off for good behavior—okay, maybe the time off was to allow the chemo to leave my system so I could start radiation therapy, but I like my excuse better. So what did I do on my spring break? The first week I rested up. The second week I started walking outside and occasionally made it through the day without a nap. And the third week, the most exciting week of all, I pulled off "the great escape," hopping a plane with Gene and flying to Texas to visit my mother and siblings!

It was a great trip filled with exciting events, like watching the TSA agent compare my driver's license photo with my current bald head. I just shrugged at him, and he said the kindest thing: "I can still tell it's you." Then the escalator at the airport was broken, so we had to climb a long flight of stairs to get to our gate. I just stuck my chin out and said, "Bring it on," and started climbing. I did pause about three-fourths of the way up and could feel the TSA agents' eyes on me. Do you think they were laying odds on whether I would make it? I know there was an elevator located next to the stairs, but that was for the elderly and disabled. I figured I was healthy enough to climb one flight of stairs. (I use cancer as an excuse only when I don't want to carry my own groceries or do certain chores.) I managed to scale the flight of stairs with only minimal panting. All this activity resulted in a nice nap on the plane.

When we landed at DFW and the doors of the plane opened, I could feel an odd phenomenon called spring! The air was warm, and the sun was shining. It was amazing. My jacket went into my bag, and I savored the feeling. We decided to celebrate our trip with a stop for lunch at Whataburger. Yum! For those of you who have never heard of it, I'm sorry for your loss. Whataburger actually puts mustard—yes, you heard me, mustard—on their hamburgers. No ketchup, no mayo, no foofy stuff. Just lettuce, pickles, and mustard. The way God intended hamburgers to be. I sat and counted off the reasons I loved my hamburger to Gene as he just grinned. Truthfully, he couldn't believe that I wasn't giving him a hard time about eating a hamburger and telling him how bad it was for him.

This was my first visit home since my father's funeral, so it was bittersweet. But my father would have been the first to tell me that I must go on. We had a wonderful visit with my mom, and we took long walks down her driveway and around her ponds twice a day. My siblings and nieces and nephews came to visit, and we had a good ol' Texas cookout on Sunday. I got priority seating in the shade and watched everyone get sunburned. But it was a beautiful day, and I sat with my hat off and let the breeze blow my…scalp? My nephew's son, age five, kept telling me to put my hat back on because "You's got no hair!" I told him I cut it off so that I could get ready faster in the mornings. It was hard to say good-bye to everyone, but I will see them in June at my son's wedding in Vegas. What a party that will be.

Now I'm home and ready to begin radiation therapy tomorrow. I will have daily radiation (yes, I said daily) for six-and-a-half weeks, and I go to chemo to receive Herceptin every three weeks. I have half a dozen other appointments in conjunction with these appointments and a calendar from hell to help me keep track of everything. I'm wondering what I did with my time before cancer. I vowed that I would not let cancer take over my life, but it does seem to for a while. A friend asked me if I got an assistant to help keep track of everything. I think this is the one patient perk they haven't thought of at the cancer center. Where is that suggestion box when you need it?

First Radiation Treatment

Friday, April 19: I had my first of thirty-three radiation treatments yesterday, and I'm just glowing! The appointment began with me meeting the technicians who will be helping me each day. They took the time to explain the equipment and explain that while I would be in the room alone at times, there were cameras and microphones in the room so they could monitor me and come assist me if I called for help. I took this as both reassuring and a caution not to do anything embarrassing, because people could be watching.

The first step in radiation is taking your clothes off from the waist up. I then had my choice of designer capes to wear. I chose the fleece one because it was bright and colorful and didn't look like a hospital gown. I quickly learned to keep a firm grip on the front of the cape as it tended to fly over my shoulder as I walked through the halls. Is it still considered flashing if you have only one breast?

The techs show me to the radiation room and point out the nice, hard radiation table. They have placed my customized form, which is monogrammed with my name in Sharpie, at the head of the table. Apparently, they made the form for me during my simulation when I wasn't paying attention. I glance at the long row of forms for other patients hanging at the back of the room. There is bound to be a joke here, but I am nervous and not sure what to expect in radiation.

I get as comfortable as possible with my hands above my head and an elastic band around my feet. The band keeps people like me from wiggling their feet during radiation. They provide nice handles for you to grip above your head. Snug as a bug, I tell you. That is, until the tech flips back the cape and exposes my chest.

They take a series of four X-rays to make sure I am lined up perfectly, and they write down a series of measurements for future use. The techs tell me my doctor is off today, so one of her partners will be coming in to verify that I'm lined up correctly. The doctor comes in and introduces himself. Now remember that I'm lying on a table with my arms above my head and a fleece cape partially covering me and obstructing my view. I have been told not to move. Because of my bifocals, I can see only a blurred image of the doctor from the nose up as he waves at me, and I chuckle. I tell him this is the strangest way I have met someone since childbirth.

Everything is set, and it is time for radiation. I'm told to breathe normally but not to move. Isn't that a contradiction? They tell me I won't feel anything and it will take only a couple of minutes. I grip the handles above my head like they are a lifeline. I feel my heart racing as the machine begins to make noise. I stare at the skylight with images of palm trees and wish I were anywhere but here. I don't feel anything, but my mind goes to places that are scary. And I hold my breath. I remember that they can see me and force myself to relax my hands and to breathe shallow breaths. I'm afraid to take deep breaths in case this makes me move closer to the radiation.

The tech tells me that the rest of my appointments will go much faster and verifies the time for my appointment the next day. I dress quickly and meet my daughter, Danielle, in the waiting room, and we leave. She asks me how it went. I can't talk. I just want out of the building. She understands immediately and starts chatting about the weather. We get in the car, and the tears start pouring down my cheeks. Danielle reaches over and holds my hand, and we sit quietly for several minutes. How did we raise such a compassionate daughter? I gather myself and say, "Shit!" and we both start laughing. She asks if it hurt, and I tell her no. This is more of a head game for me.

Ever since I was diagnosed, I have wanted to avoid radiation. My husband is surprised by this. He tells me that most people want to get out of chemo and don't mind radiation. It would be hard to put into words all my fears about radiation, but I will list a couple. I'm afraid of the damage it can cause and the permanence of that damage. In chemo, if you start to get too sick, they stop the chemo. In radiation, the damage doesn't show up for a while. My other fear is that I have known people who had too much exposure to radiation and died from it. I realize that medicine has come a long way since the early days and that if I understand it better, it will lessen my fears. So I will talk with my doctor and work my way through this.

In the meantime, today is a fun day filled with radiation and chemo. A doubleheader! The way I see it, that gives me twice the number of techs and nurses to give a hard time!

Kamikaze Corner

Monday, April 22: Each time I exit the interstate to go to chemo or radiation, I have to travel through an intersection that I call Kamikaze Corner. It is the corner where the highway off-ramp meets the street and there is a four-way stop. For some reason, people constantly run the stop signs and have near misses or collisions. The city has even gone to the trouble of adding red flags on the stop signs to try to attract drivers' attention. And one inspired business owner has set up a collision center on the opposite corner to rake in the business.

On weeks when I have a driver, I always warn them about this intersection, and yet three of my friends have been guilty of running the stop sign even after the warning. So I have a new strategy. I have started taking my hat off before I get to this intersection in hopes of the sun's reflection off my shiny, bald head grabbing other drivers' attention and causing them to slow down. If nothing else, I'm hoping that when they nearly run into me, the fact that they nearly hit a *cancer patient* on her way to treatment will shame them. I try to look suitably ill as well. The guilt may send a few people into therapy. Hmm. Maybe I can set up a counseling corner across from the collision center!

Pasties

Tuesday, April 23: I think the lack of a breast on one side is starting to bug my doctor and the techs, because they keep putting decorations on my chest. First it was tattoos, and then yesterday and today they gave me pasties. The tech showed them to me and claimed they were devices to measure the intensity of the radiation I'm receiving, but the clear stickers they left on overnight kind of look like smiley faces. I told Gene they were for good behavior. He snickered. Thirty years of marriage and he knows better.

I did learn some new things in the past few days. I have decided to limit my questions to the techs to two a day. That way I won't become a nuisance, and it helps to pass the time. I have learned that the reason you can't wear deodorant or lotion while receiving radiation is because it could increase the irritation to the skin. I have been given special deodorant and lotion to use. (It is nice to know that I'm special.) Both come in spray bottles, which I find interesting. I have never had lotion in a spray bottle before. I can tell you that the deodorant does not have an antiperspirant in it.

I have also learned that the doctors calculate tolerances in your radiation levels to allow for breathing, so I can breathe without fear of being too close to the machine. And the snap on the gown will not get hot under radiation.

And finally, my favorite question of all. On my first treatment, I noticed a button on the speaker in the ceiling, and I swear it said "call" on it. I asked one of the techs if it really was a call button and how on earth I was supposed to push it. She tilted her head back and looked up, and sure enough, it was a call button. She said that no one had mentioned it before. Leave it to me! She promised they could hear me without me pushing the button, and I suspect that if I tried to stand on the metal table, they would be in the room in less than twenty seconds. Don't you think the installer was laughing as he installed that speaker? I'm so tempted to get one of those extendable pointers that teachers use and push that button to see what happens.

Getting to the Bottom of Things

Friday, April 26: Let's face it. I have never been good at doing things just because someone tells me to. I want to know why and how things work. And the response that makes me most crazy is, "Because we have always done it this way." That is like waving a big red flag in front of me. I generally make it my mission to get that policy changed. Kind of like the no-nail-polish rule for surgery. I painted my middle toes just for the heck of it and as a statement.

So it shouldn't surprise you that I decided to get a better look at the treatment table yesterday. Each visit, the techs tell me to lie still, and they pull and shove and twist and turn the table underneath me until the laser pointers line up with the tattoos on my chest and ribs. Being the helpful sort, I always try to help them move me, and they have to remind me to let them do the work. I have nothing but time to lie there and wonder how this table works, so I decided to take a closer look at it after my treatment. (For my friends Barb and Tess, who have seen me crawl under things at parties just to see how they worked, yes, I was thinking of you. But these people have video monitors, and I was sure I would get caught. So I asked permission to look under the table.)

From the hips down, the table is stationary. The middle section, under the ribs, moves from left to right. And the top section, under the head and shoulders, swivels in a semicircle. Pretty cool! The techs call out numbers like 91.3 and 86.5 to help line me up. I asked them where they find those numbers, and they told me they are reflecting off my chest. Cool again! I'm tempted to slip a mirror in my pocket so I can see for myself.

Please note that at no point did I touch the radiation equipment. I promise. I state this because a couple hours after I left, the tech called me to say that the equipment was broken and they needed to reschedule my appointment time for the next day. And today, while I was there, one of the light bulbs burned out on the equipment, which meant I had to move to yet another room while maintenance fixed it. I promise it wasn't my fault. All I did was look.

Brittany, my tech, offered to go into the waiting room and tell Gene what was going on. I asked her to lead with, "It isn't Kathy's fault, but…"

The Way People Treat You

Friday, May 3: One of my observations has been about the way people treat you when you have cancer. It fascinates me that I feel the same, but people treat me differently. In the early stages, people would hug me like I was fragile or like my chest must hurt. I would tell them to "hug me like you mean it." Breast cancer doesn't hurt.

Once you lose your hair, all bets are off. It is hard to go unnoticed. When you are out in public, people tend to go one of two ways. Either they can't look you in the eye, or they treat you really, really nicely. I have had the best service at restaurants since becoming bald. I kid you not. My water glass is never empty. I seem to get served extra-large portions. If I pull my jacket around my shoulders, the manager turns up the heat in the restaurant. I watched my ice melt and Gene and the other customers sweat bullets at one restaurant until I finally relented and removed my jacket.

Another observation is that people let you cut in line. They don't just let you; they practically beg you to. I find it amusing. And as long as I'm bald, I will never have to carry my own groceries. I'm telling you, a less respectable person could really take advantage of this cancer thing.

When my mom was here, she commented that no one would even know I had cancer except for the bald head and missing eyebrows and eyelashes. I cocked my head, thought about it, and tried not to laugh. I'm sure there was a compliment in there somewhere.

I think the best advice I got was from my two mentors, Julie and Chris. Early on, they told me that my job was to take care of myself, to do what made me comfortable, and to let everyone else get over it. I didn't fully understand that at first, but over time, I have understood what they are talking about. Wear a wig if you want to. Wear a hat or go bald if that is what you want. Wear your prosthetic or not. Get creative with scarves or jackets, or just accept that your temporary breasts aren't level.

Since I can't wear my prosthetic breast during radiation, I'm dealing with that last one daily. I wear a camisole with a pocket that holds quilt batting on one side, and I sag on the other side. As mentioned previously, Gene and Danielle have devised a signal for "your breast is on your shoulder" that has me rearranging now and then. We just laugh as I shift and adjust. Nice to know they have my back (or front!).

Mileposts

Tuesday, May 7: My dear, sweet husband knows how much I like to set mileposts or goals along a long journey to mark my progress. I'm a chronic list maker, and my favorite thing to do is to mark things off the list when I complete them. My friends tease me about this, but I find it cathartic.

Gene has helped me blow up pumpkins in phase one of chemo, release balloons in phase two, and brainstorm for ideas for radiation. I just couldn't think of a good milepost that wasn't too much work yet was significant and fun. I kept getting stumped trying to imagine something that was legal and safe and yet resembled a mushroom cloud after a nuclear explosion. Even with my creative thinking, nothing came to mind!

So Gene came up with the idea of building me a carnival-type shooting gallery that we could hang balloons on and shoot at. Now I realize there appears to be a lot of shooting involved with my recovery. I should mention that I'm not a big fan of guns. They hold no interest for me. I neither approve nor disapprove of them. I just don't care to shoot them. But I do like blowing things up. So when Gene put this activity together, he assured me that all I would have to do was shoot a BB gun, and I would get to blow up balloons. (And it seems a lot safer than nuclear explosions!)

Each week, we inflate five balloons to represent the five sessions of radiation and hang them on a pole. Then we take turns shooting at the balloons. Nobody gets hurt, and we have a lot of laughs with the exercise. I actually popped two balloons with one shot the other day.

Amazing Grace

Saturday, May 11: The cancer center I go to is an affiliate of Mercy Hospital, and they share a public address system. During the course of treatment, you hear trauma alerts and general announcements. One of the fun announcements is when a new baby is born. A soft lullaby is played every time a mother delivers a baby at the hospital. You can't help but smile when you hear it. I often spend a moment thinking of my own three children's deliveries.

Yesterday, while I was waiting for radiation, I heard a familiar song and then I realized it was "Amazing Grace." I frowned and thought, "Surely they don't play that every time they lose a patient." How depressing that could be for the other patients. Then I realized that the music wasn't coming from the speaker but from the lobby. I walked out and saw a violinist softly playing music.

Now before you all start throwing darts at me, I do know that "Amazing Grace" is played other than at funerals. But let's face it: it is played at a lot of funerals. It always makes me cry. So I entertained myself on the way home coming up with a new playlist for the violinist:

- "We Gotta Get Out of This Place"
- "Stayin' Alive"
- "Save Me"
- "Help!"
- "Walk On By"
- "I Will Survive"
- "I Won't Give Up"
- "Still Not over You"
- "Movin' On"
- "Faith"
- "Hold On"
- "Stand by Me"

Halfway

Monday, May 13: I just passed the halfway mark of radiation treatments by finishing my eighteenth treatment today. To celebrate, my X-ray team broke out the Magic Markers and drew on my chest—again. However, this time they used a green marker. Since I hadn't used up my two questions for the day, I asked if each type of treatment was color coded. And sure enough, they are! Black is used for CT scans, and green is used for "bonus" treatments. I know they use purple in the operating room, so I keep a keen eye out for purple markers.

My bonus treatments involve a very targeted treatment to the scar area from my mastectomy. The tech tells me that they have found that breast cancer tends to recur first in this area, so they like to give it extra attention for my last five treatments. The fact that someone is even talking about "my last five treatments" is exciting to me. The finish line is attainable!

So today, the radiologist channeled her inner child and wrote all over my chest with a green marker. It isn't like you can't see the scar without highlighting it, so I'm not sure why the marker was necessary. But she drew a large green rectangle on my chest, and then the techs traced it onto a thin piece of plastic to use for my treatment. I was told I could bathe as usual, the marker would wear off, and they would redraw the area in my final treatments. Super. I can't wait. But I'm going to ask them to use a checkered pattern on my last treatment to represent the finish line.

Supervision

Tuesday, May 14: When I first met with my radiologist, I asked if I would be able to go with Gene to Palm Springs in May. She told me that it was too many days off from radiation, so I could not go with him. I was upset. Gene is getting to go someplace cool, and I'm getting left at home. I fully intended to pout all week, but Gene suggested I invite Steven home for the week to keep me company.

I really think that Gene wanted Steven to be here to supervise me. I tend to get into trouble when left to my own devices for very long. I don't mean to get into trouble. It's just that some things seem like good ideas when I start them and turn out to be bad ideas later. But seriously—having Steven supervise? He has the same sense of humor that I do and is equally creative. We both tend to get into trouble when we are bored. I have a grin on my face just thinking about a week with a playmate. Gene looked seriously worried when I asked him to pick up some exploding targets for me.

Radiation Myths

Thursday, May 16: I have been honing my interrogation skills by asking my radiation team questions during each treatment. Slowly but surely I have been dispensing with some of the radiation myths and fears I have on my mind. Before you read further, let me remind you that if you are using this book for scientific or medical information, you are in trouble. These are simply my observations and interpretations. Whew! The disclaimer is out of the way and gives me deniability. Tess, my friend and attorney, would be so proud!

The first myth I heard was that you are actually radioactive during radiation. Nope, not true for my type of radiation treatments. But wouldn't it be cool if you were? I wasn't really worried about this one and suspected it wasn't true, but it sure seemed like a good excuse to get out of things I didn't want to do anyway. There are some types of radiation treatment that can make you radioactive, but those aren't the type I am having.

Next, I was told I would not be able to go out into the sun while I was having radiation treatments. Again, not true. But that one did have my anxiety level up. Due to my treatments, I missed fall and endured winter. I sure didn't want to miss spring. I do have to keep the radiated area covered. But it was my chest, and I had no plans to bare it anyway.

I nearly had a meltdown when someone told me I would not be able to take baths. That one has some truth to it. I'm asked to shower every other day and to limit myself to one short lukewarm bath per week if I want a bath. This is to help keep my skin from drying out and getting more irritated. I've been instructed to use no bath gels or oils and only mild soap, please. Well, mark my chart "noncompliant," because a short lukewarm bath is just not acceptable. Long baths are my sanctuary. I do limit myself to one bath a week, but the water is warm, and I'm not getting out till it is cold. And I may fudge that every-other-day shower rule now and then.

My doctor and I had a long discussion today about why they need to take photos of my chest and who has access to those photos. I was assured that only limited staff have access to that portion of my medical records. I explained to the doctor that this freaks me out, but she assured me the photos were safe. When the tech took my photo today, she showed me the image, and I could see that my face wasn't visible. This does reassure me quite a bit, but I still don't like it.

One of my more interesting and ongoing discussions with my team is regarding radiation exposure. All our lives we have been told to limit exposure to X-rays and that too many can give you cancer. Well, I already have cancer, so shouldn't we limit it even more? Even the dentist covers up your important areas when he takes X-rays, and the dental assistants leave the room. My techs explained to me that when you get normal X-rays, they are using low doses of radiation, and this causes "scatter" to other exposed areas. In radiation therapy, they use high doses of radiation, so there is less scatter. So here is my question: if it is so safe, why do the techs still leave the room? Ha! It would just be mean-spirited to ask, so I'm going to keep that one to myself.

I still chuckle to myself when they tell me to "lie still and breathe normally." Right, like that is ever going to happen. Since I haven't figured a way to get out of radiation, and my mind goes to crazy places during radiation, I have developed ways to entertain myself and stay occupied. I get radiation treatments from two different angles and at two different levels, totaling four treatments each day. I started out trying to count how many seconds each of the treatments lasted and wondering why they all aren't the same length. That got boring after a couple of weeks, so now I'm practicing to see how long I can hold my breath. You never know when that skill might come in handy.

Changes

Friday, May 24: You cannot go through this disease (cancer) without changing. At some point, you stop to consider your own mortality and what effect you have had on the world, your friends, and your family. What will you do if you survive? What will you do if you realize you have only a short time left? Will you face the disease with courage, or fear, or resignation, or humor? None of us knows how we will react until we go through the diagnosis and treatment.

I know that I have changed. I'm already thinking about the things I will or won't do after treatment. I have decided I won't stress over the little things. I went to get a pedicure today and was asked to pick a color. I stewed over my decision, then turned to Danielle and said, "Surprise me." I now have blue toenails, and they make me laugh. I would never have picked this color of polish, but what does it hurt? I'm sure my radiology team will get a kick out of it.

When the chemo effects had me so tired I could barely function, I discovered that if you leave the clean dishes in the dishwasher for a day, they are still clean! And despite what my mother told me, if you don't make your bed one day, it doesn't go on your permanent record. So I am not going to worry if I fail to unload the dishwasher.

I won't attend another meeting that doesn't have a purpose. Give me something productive to do, or stay off my calendar!

I will enjoy a beautiful day. I get outside every chance I get and tilt my face toward the sky and thank God that I'm upright and not nauseated. When people ask me how I'm doing, I grin and say, "I'm super. How are you?"

I will continue to travel and explore new places and take on new challenges. I will hug my children tightly every opportunity that I get. I will thank Gene every chance I get and hold his hand when he walks beside me. And when I tell someone I will pray for them, I will mean it and I won't forget.

Please don't think I'm changing the essence of who I am. I will still be ornery and poke fun at the world. When I first lost my hair, I said I would never complain about a bad hair day again. I already know that was a big fat lie! But I do plan to have some fun as my hair grows out and try some new hairstyles. I'm thinking short, spiky hair could be fun for a while.

It will be interesting to see what other changes come into my life. Stay tuned.

Boost Radiation

Thursday, May 30: My X-ray techs told me that my last five radiation treatments would be boost treatments to the scar area. I said okay because I really couldn't even come up with a question at the time. I called Tess, who is a former X-ray tech, and asked what "boost" meant. She said she didn't know but it couldn't be good. We died laughing.

Since then, I have learned a bit more about boost. The definition of boost radiation is, apparently, an excuse to use more Sharpies on the patient. It is also a good excuse to add more attachments to the radiation machine.

For the past two mornings, my team has drawn dots on my chest with a green Sharpie. I'm not talking three or four dots. I have twenty-six green dots circling my chest. Yes, I counted them. They tend to rub off on the underside of my shirt. I think that is so I have something to remember after treatment ends.

A large extension is added to the radiation equipment and lowered to my chest. The extension looks like a science project made of spare dental parts. I suspect the extension is to ensure only the scar area is treated. I'm almost afraid to ask. One arm is behind my head, and I am asked to turn my head to the side. It is a silly pose, and I find myself smiling. Sort of, "Look at me. I'm a topless model!"

After the dots are lined up with the machine, things go quickly. I count about twenty seconds for the treatment, and then I'm done. I have only three more treatments to go, so I bounce out of the cancer center and take a fresh look around. And that's when I notice it: the special parking places for radiation patients. Are you kidding me? I have been going to radiation for six weeks, and I just now noticed there is special parking for me? I have been parking with the "regular" cancer patients all this time. In fact, I have been parking in the furthest spots because I feel stronger now that chemo is only every three weeks. I could have had front-row parking! Call me Miss Observant.

The Drive

Friday, May 31: For the past six weeks, I have driven into town each day for radiation treatments. Five days a week. Thirty-five miles each way. I have watched the fields turn green and the trees leaf out. I have watched rain, tractors tilling and planting fields, flooding, more rain, and wild turkeys courting. As entertaining as all of these things are, they still aren't enough to keep my brain occupied. So I have found my own amusement along the way.

I like to make up stories about where people are going. If someone has a Florida license plate, I wonder if they really drove all the way from Florida. I imagine myself making that long trip. My husband's dream vacation is a cross-country driving trip. That is my nightmare vacation. I start banging my head on the headrest at about five hours into a trip, which always makes him laugh. Traveling with the kids was never the limiting factor for us. Traveling with me is. I want out of the car. I want to "do something." So this monotonous trip back and forth to town daily is making me crazy.

Some days, I take my hat off and count the number of double takes I get when people pass me. I try not to laugh when they attempt to be subtle about it. I wonder what is going through their minds. What follows, "Oh, she has cancer"? Is it "Thank God it isn't me" or "Doesn't she have a nice, smooth head?" or "My, look how incredibly young she looks!" or, better yet, "Maybe I should slow down."

Other days, I crank up the radio and sing along. It should be noted that I never know the words to a song, and I don't let that bother me. I just make up words to follow the melody. It helps me think. I know it seems strange, but I get some of my best ideas and creative thinking done while singing along to music. Somehow it releases my creativity. People pass me and grin back at me as I smile and sing along.

On bad days, when my chest is so sore and my brain is telling me that it is crazy to go in and have more radiation, I call Tess, and she talks me into town. She is that person who I can laugh with and cry with, often at the same time. As a former X-ray tech, she understands why I don't want to go to radiation. She promises to support me if I decide to quit, but she also says that if I quit and she supports me and I die, she will never forgive herself. This always makes me laugh. Finally, someone who just puts it out there! I usually spend a couple minutes on the phone with her, sitting in the parking lot and looking at the cancer clinic. She always ends the call with some ridiculous suggestion about radiation that has me laughing hysterically as I enter the clinic. God put Tess in my life for so many reasons, but I appreciate her humor most of all.

Only two more days of radiation and then I'm only left with phase three of chemo, tamoxifen, and reconstruction if possible. I plan to ring the bell loudly on Tuesday.

Radiation Fatigue

Saturday, June 1: Prior to starting radiation, I heard a lot about the fatigue you get toward the end of treatment. That confused me. I understand why you can get fatigued with chemotherapy. After all, they are putting lots of toxins in you that can lower your blood counts. But why would radiation cause fatigue? I asked my husband, my doctor, and my techs about it, and they all answered the same: no one really knows why. It just happens.

I experienced my share of fatigue during chemo, so I wasn't looking forward to it with radiation. If memory serves me, one particularly bad weekend day, I slept nearly twenty out of twenty-four hours. Fortunately, I didn't have any problem with radiation fatigue until the last week of treatment. I remember when it hit. I woke up one morning and got out of bed and thought, "Whoa. I'm exhausted, and I need to go back to bed." Unfortunately, I couldn't go back to bed because I had to get ready to go to radiation. Ironic, isn't it?

Radiation fatigue is different from normal fatigue and chemo fatigue in that rest doesn't help. I could take a nap and wake up exhausted. It is like being in a perpetual Dramamine fog. My doctor recommends that I take a walk outside when I get too tired. Dolly Dog and I have done many laps on the mile-long driveway. But the mosquitoes are having a field day with all the recent flooding, and I'm in fear of getting West Nile virus next. Dolly has been vaccinated against West Nile. I have not. So now we are working on inside projects. I do most of the work, and Dolly Dog provides security.

Epic Monday

Monday, June 3: For months, there have been whispers in the halls at the cancer clinic about the transition to a new electronic medical records system called Epic. It was spoken of with fear and apprehension. Nurses would put a brave face on and say that it was supposed to be much better than the current system, but I could see fear in their eyes. They weren't fooling me. I named the transition day Epic Monday.

So as the big day approached, signs went up and schedulers tried to avoid having patients come in on Epic Monday. Unfortunately, since radiation appointments were daily, I had an appointment on the dreaded day. The techs handed me a piece of paper explaining what was going on and requested that I show up fifteen minutes early. I'm always there fifteen minutes early, so no problem?

As I arrived at the building, things appeared to be normal. I checked the third-floor windows for cracks or nurses preparing to jump, but everything seemed fine. I walked into the building to see dozens of people wearing orange construction vests. This made me chuckle. I love it when someone goes with a theme. I walked into the radiation area and asked, "Is everyone okay?" and they laughed. Registration was easy, and nothing bad happened. I was offered a cookie for my patience. I got a new photo taken for my file, which was okay with me since I now have a hint of hair. Radiation went without a hitch, and I left for the day thinking that was much ado about nothing.

Fast-forward to Wednesday and my research appointment. Once again, I am asked to sign in, but there seems to be some confusion and discussion about a wristband. They decide I don't need one and send me to the waiting area. My research nurse comes out to get me and asks if I'm okay. She tells me that the computer says I have been down in radiation for the past forty-seven hours. Oh heck no! I spend as little time there as I can. My nurse says, "Why didn't you call us? We would have come and helped you escape!" They take me back to the infusion area for my injection, and there is another discussion about a wristband. I'm all alone in a "special" area, and people in orange vests walk by and say, "Oh, you are the special one." Yup. That's me.

"Special" in this case means "We don't know what to do with you. And why aren't you wearing a wristband? Our new computer system has no idea what to do with you either. And by the way, Epic says that you are still in radiation." I sort of sat back and let the orange vests deal with it since I figured I would only get in the way. I did offer to take a stab at the new computer system and help them figure it out. I'm fearless at a computer, which occasionally results in trouble.

I had time to eat a banana, drink a soft drink, read and sign an updated research consent form, make a few new friends, and talk to a few nurses. Everyone kept apologizing, but it was quite entertaining. When I finally left, I looked over my shoulder and told them not to forget to sign me out of radiation. Snicker.

I'm Done with That!

Tuesday, June 4: Today was my last day of radiation. Thirty-three treatments done! Six-and-a-half weeks, 2,310 miles in round trips on my SUV, one holiday, ten doctor's appointments, three chemo appointments, two research appointments, one genetic appointment, thirty-three "You can do its" and "I'm proud of yous" from Mom, nine support phone calls to Tess, and seven massages. But who is counting? Done, done, done. I was so excited to leave today that I nearly missed my free massage that comes with radiation treatments. I made it to the end and completed radiation treatment. Woo-hoo!

I didn't ring the bell today. It sort of got lost in the shuffle of my running out of the building. Maybe it jingled a little as I rushed past it. My radiation team did give me a single, perfect red rose and told me they enjoyed treating me. That is better than ringing a bell, because they seemed sincere in the gesture. I was touched. How difficult must it be for them to face cancer each day, knowing that they can't save everyone? Yet they remain positive and interested in their patients. We talked about our weekends and the weather, how bad the flooding would be, kids and dogs, my new shoes, and sometimes about radiation. They teased me about being fifteen minutes early every day. They answered my questions and always met me with a smile. I grin each time I walk by the rose, and stop and take a smell.

When I first started radiation and was first handed my appointment calendar, I remember thinking I didn't have time for radiation. Seriously. Who has time to drive over an hour each day for a fifteen-minute appointment? Now I wonder what I will do with my mornings. Maybe Dolly Dog and I will double our walking time. And maybe I will return to work. But first, I'm going to use the time to get ready for my son's wedding in twelve days. As a final celebration of the end of radiation, Gene and I are going to blow up a watermelon this weekend. Now all that is left is phase three of chemo and tamoxifen.

How to Kill a Watermelon

Friday, June 14: As I leave radiation on my last day, I stop at the grocery store to pick up a few things. Just inside the door is a large stand of ripe watermelons. "Hmm," I think. "Wouldn't that be fun to blow up?" So I grab one (and two more just for the fun of it) and put them in my cart. I feel frustration management therapy in my future. The watermelons roll from side to side in the back of my SUV as I make the thirty-mile trip home, but I laugh each time they *thunk* on the side of the car. I cross my fingers that they don't split and leak sticky juice all over my vehicle. When I get home, I line them up on the bench next to the door in the garage.

When Gene gets home, he walks in and says, "I take it we are going to blow up some more stuff to celebrate the end of radiation." You can't get much past this man I am married to! He is a good sport and stops in town to purchase the Tannerite. What did we do for entertainment before my brother-in-law introduced us to this stuff?

As I have mentioned in the past, I'm not a fan of shooting, but I get such a kick out of watching something blow up. In addition, my right shoulder is very sore and oozing from the radiation treatment. The thought of having a rifle hit it is unbearable. Fortunately, Gene is willing to take one for the team. We hear a neighbor target-practicing in the woods. I joke that I bet we can make more noise than he makes. Gene lines up his shot and *BOOM!* There is a flash, and watermelon debris, juice, and smoke go everywhere. I can barely hold the camera still because I'm laughing so hard. There is total silence from the neighbor, and Gene and I laugh harder. I love this man!

Radiation Side Effects

Wednesday, June 26: During radiation, my biggest concern was whether my skin would be healed before I attended my son's wedding. Unfortunately, it was not. I had what I have heard called a "wet reaction." The skin on my chest and under my armpit blistered, cracked, oozed, and peeled for two-and-a-half weeks. The pain was significant. I wore a flannel cape around the house to give my chest as much air as possible. At night, I wore my husband's T-shirts to try to absorb most of the mess. The dry air in Las Vegas and time helped to dry out the skin.

Wouldn't you know that I would get selected for a pat-down on our return trip to home. I looked at the TSA agent with pleading eyes and said, "Be very careful." She was very considerate. Chalk up one more perk for being practically bald.

At three weeks, the last crack has healed, and most of the peeling has stopped. The skin looks much better, and I'm using cocoa butter to soften it and make it more pliable. I will always have to protect this skin and keep it out of the sun, so that means a T-shirt over my swimsuit. I can live with that.

In an earlier post, I talked about radiation fatigue. I don't know why I had it in my head that the fatigue would go away in about two weeks. Probably because I knew that was the extent of my attention span. Unfortunately, I'm three weeks out of radiation, and I'm still fatigued. Since I don't have a follow-up appointment for another week, I went to my favorite website to see what they said about the topic. Sadly, they say that radiation fatigue can last six weeks to a year, and in some cases, years. This does not fit into my schedule.

Nope. I'm not having it. I have officially run out of patience for side effects and being sick. I don't know how much mind over matter works for medical issues, but if sheer willpower works, I'm going to eliminate "I'm so tired" from my vocabulary. So today I started my new training program. I took Dolly Dog for her usual morning walk, but I stepped it up a notch. I marched down the driveway swinging my arms high. Then I did the goose step back to the house. (Good thing our nearest neighbor needs binoculars to see me!) Dolly kept looking at me and cocking her head to try to figure out what was wrong with me. When I got back to the house, I turned around and walked backward down the drive again. Dolly kept looking over her shoulder to see what I was looking at.

Later, Gene called to say he couldn't make it home for lunch, but he wanted to make sure that I ate something. I was so tired by that point that I heated up a cup of soup and then fell facedown on the sofa for a nap. I need to learn moderation!

.

CHAPTER 6
CHEMOTHERAPY PHASE THREE

Phase Three of Chemo

Wednesday, June 13, 2013: Phase three of my treatment started in April and is a single drug called Herceptin. It is given every three weeks through my port like my other chemo meds. Herceptin isn't really a chemotherapy drug. It is an antibody that interferes with the HER2/neu receptor. HER2/neu can cause cancer to reproduce uncontrollably. So when I got my pathology report after my biopsy, I was told that I was HER2/neu positive and would need additional treatment to contain and prevent my cancer from coming back. One of my nurses told me to think of this phase as chemo maintenance. I like that. "Maintenance" doesn't sound as scary as "chemo."

I have had a couple of days when I had radiation and chemo maintenance on the same day, which makes for a lot of running around at the cancer clinic. It is at times like these that I am so glad I go to a cancer clinic where everything is within the same building: sort of a one-stop shop. And since their medical records are all integrated, if I get hung up somewhere and don't show up on time, the staff can find where I am in the building. I find these combined appointments amusing. I go from one check-in desk to another and ask, "Where am I supposed to be next?" I do have a master calendar, but I feel like a freshman on the first day of school walking around looking at the calendar and then looking up to see where I am.

The good news about phase three is that most of the side effects are gone, and it takes far less time than other phases. Not only that, but I can drive myself home because I'm not having to take the premeds that made me so tired. The only premed I have to take is Tylenol, and my infusion lasts only thirty minutes. I feel like such a big girl getting to go to my appointments by myself! If all goes well, I can be in and out of chemo, labs, and doctor visit in two hours. What will I do with my spare time? Phase three of chemo lasts until January 2014.

Genetic Testing

Thursday, May 30: There has been a lot of talk about genetic testing for breast cancer since Angelina Jolie came out with the news that she had preventative mastectomies after testing positive for BRCA1. Now everyone is wondering if they should be tested and asking if I was tested. Let me just say that this isn't a test you get lightly. You and your physician can decide if the test is necessary and discuss what the results could mean. It is a very expensive test, and insurance may not cover it unless you have a significant family history to warrant the test.

When my doctors learned that my dad's three sisters had breast cancer, they recommended I visit with a genetic counselor. We sat down and did a family tree listing the family members, the ages and reasons of death for those who were deceased, and any cancers for those living. This included my grandparents and parents and their siblings, cousins, nieces, and nephews. At this point, the counselor determined I was a candidate for genetic testing. We then submitted the family tree to my insurance for consideration of coverage for the $4,000 test.

From a procedure standpoint, genetic testing is very easy. It can be done with either a cheek swab or blood test. I chose to have a blood test as it can be more accurate. My blood was then shipped to a lab, and I was told it would take at least three weeks to get my results. It took a bit longer than that, and my counselor called today to tell me that I was both BRCA1 and BRCA2 negative and that there weren't any abnormal mutations of my genes. So my cancer was "just one of those things" that happens in life. I can live with that.

Had I tested positive, I would then need to have a conversation with my siblings, mother, and children as to whether they should be tested. My doctor also explained that if I tested positive, we would need to discuss having my ovaries removed as I would also be at risk for ovarian cancer. As you can imagine, a positive result can open a big can of worms and affect not only your life but other people's lives as well. I knew and accepted these possibilities prior to being tested. The one thing that persuaded me to do the testing was a statement from my daughter. She said, "The greatest gift you could give us all would be to be tested and get a negative report." Fortunately, that is exactly what happened.

The Wedding

Sunday, June 30: On June 17, my son Nicholas married Samantha, the love of his life. It was a beautiful, simple ceremony in Las Vegas with two dozen family and friends in attendance. The day started with my siblings and I taking our mother to breakfast and then out to teach her to gamble. We don't often get together, so it is always special when we do get the chance. And we had so many laughs as we taught Mom how to feed the one-armed bandits.

Later that morning, Sam's mom and Danielle and I had a Vegas makeup artist do our hair and makeup. Who knew that there would be so many layers of makeup and so many questions? I was so out of my element, but fortunately Danielle was there to answer any questions. Francesca, the makeup artist, penciled on eyebrows and glued on eyelashes, and I looked in the mirror and saw a hint of my former self.

We lunched and laughed and celebrated the day as Nick and his friends played card games on the floor of the suite overlooking the Strip. It was casual. It was fun. It was how a wedding day should be. We laughed as Nick had to keep running up and down the elevator to pick up the cake, the flowers, the photographer. We all agreed that living with a key card–controlled elevator was just not our style!

Watching Sam's mom helping her dress was a special moment. I felt privileged to get a peek into that window. And as I looked at my son, grown and about to start on a new chapter in his life, I could see so much of his father: a kindness and concern for others, a deep sense of responsibility, a friend for life. And sweet Sam, we couldn't have picked a better daughter-in-law.

I watched as Sam pinned a rose to Nick's lapel and thought of so many things I would like to tell them. Mostly I wanted to tell them that I could not wish more for them than what I have found with Gene. That I hoped that thirty years from now, they could look at each other and see a friend, a lover, someone who would laugh at them and with them, someone who would hold them when they cried, and most importantly, someone who would walk with them through life's journey. Someone who would make this journey easier. But the words stuck in my throat. I said a silent prayer to God thanking him that I got to live to see this day.

Nick and Sam were married in the same church that my in-laws were married in and used my in-law's wedding rings. I didn't cry, which is a miracle since I cry at every wedding. I was quite simply happy to be alive.

Vegas, Baby!

Sunday, June 23: It would take too long to describe my eventful trip to

Vegas, but I will share some highlights.

My son's wedding was sweet and touching. I feel so thankful that I got to live to see one of my children get married and to a beautiful woman whom we adore.

Sam's (my new daughter-in-law) mom and I decided not to do the "in-law thing." We are going to be co-mothers instead.

Rachel (the bad wig) did not show up. Raquel (the good wig) cooperated until the end, when I wasn't feeling well and Gene pulled her off my head. Too funny.

Danielle commented that Vegas is good for any personal insecurities you might have, because no one is ever looking at you, as there is always someone weirder walking around.

My siblings and I decided to teach Mom how to feed the one-armed bandits (slot machines). What machine does my brother pick to teach her on? Sex in the City! It was so much fun that I texted Sam to say I might be late for hair and makeup.

My mom is a master gardener and fell in love with all the flower displays. I threatened to get a T-shirt for her that read, "If lost, find me in the Bellagio arboretum."

We took my mom on driving trips to the Hoover Dam and Red Rock Canyon. I slept through both trips. It was 113 degrees. I love air conditioning.

I got a fortune cookie that read, "Your finances are about to change for the better." It was right. I quit gambling and didn't lose any more money.

You know you have been in Vegas too long when a thirty-five-dollar burger sounds cheap.

My son's new family is wonderful. He will have lots of new aunts and uncles and cousins to get to know better. They were all very warm and supportive of the newlyweds.

The thirty-six-hour trip from hell back home was not funny. Spending an entire thirty-six-dollar American Airlines food voucher on Starbucks granola bars? Priceless!

The Trip from Hell

Monday, July 1: I love to travel. I always have. Even with the headaches that sometimes come with flying, I cannot wait to get to the airport and board a plane. I have had my share of canceled flights, lost luggage, rude passengers, and disgruntled employees, but I remained excited about travel—until my return trip from the wedding. The short version is that we experienced reservation changes, mechanical failure, incompetent or unhelpful gate agents, medical issues, overbooking, luggage issues, and weather. I was looking for locusts (pestilence) by the time we got home.

I admit that I have a policy not to write when I'm mad. Nothing good comes from writing in anger. So it has taken a while to find the humor in our travel experience and compose my letter to the airline. Here is the letter I sent to the airline:

I booked our flights to Vegas about four months in advance because I wanted to connect in Dallas and have my mother join us on the connecting flight to and from Vegas. She hasn't flown much in the past fifteen years, so we wanted to make sure she was comfortable. We encountered the usual delays and gate changes on the flight to Vegas, but things went relatively smoothly. The night before our return home, I pulled up our updated schedule online and saw that the airline had moved Gene, Danielle, and me to a different flight than Mom. How is that possible without a phone call? We decided to arrive at the airport at 8:00 a.m. in plenty of time to fix this.

Step 1. The helpful agent trying to move the line along tells me that I have to check in on a computer. I explain the issue with our tickets, and he helpfully tells me that it will cost seventy-five dollars per person for us to move back to our original flight. I'm not paying. I didn't change the flight in the first place, so I'm drawing a line in the sand.

Step 2. The agent checking our luggage says she can't help me but to check with the gate agent.

Step 3. The gate agent tells me they aren't working my flight yet and to come back an hour before the flight. I stand my ground and explain the circumstances, but since I don't have a copy of my original flight schedule on me, she says it will be seventy-five dollars per person and the flight is full, so not likely to happen. Mom states that she is a big girl and can take the flight on her own. We aren't happy, but this will at least get her into DFW at a reasonable time. We wave to Mom as she gets on her plane. She is amazed to sit down and have a vacant seat beside her, in front of her, and several more empty seats on the plane. So much for a full flight.

Step 4. My phone rings, and I start getting notices that our 1:10 p.m. flight is delayed. It continues to ring with delay notices until I get a message that we will now miss our connecting flight to Iowa and an agent would be calling me. No agent called. Ever.

Step 5. At 2:00 p.m., we find a helpful gate agent, who looks in the computer and tells us that due to mechanical issues, we have been rebooked through Denver on a 3:40 p.m. United flight and will get home about midnight. I sigh and say, "Thank you. This way I won't miss chemo tomorrow." I'm being nice. It isn't the gate agent's fault. The agent gives us new tickets and tells us that she cannot assign seats for United and that we should go to the United terminal and get the gate agent to give us seat assignments. She says they will attempt to find our luggage and move it to the United flight. What color is our luggage? Black. So we are pretty sure they will never find it.

Step 6. We find our United gate, and I approach the counter for seat assignments. The helpful agent tells us he isn't working our flight yet. Being practically bald is not helping me today. An hour later, I approach the counter, and the agent tells me the flight is full and they don't have seats for us. Would I like to go back to American or wait to see if they have some no-shows?

At this point, someone in our party decides to be a poor sport. I'm not naming names, but it isn't Gene and it isn't me. I start laughing because there doesn't seem to be anything else to do. When no seats are available, we are told to go back to American because "This is their problem, not ours." We ask about our luggage. They tell us it is going to Denver without us. We don't live in Denver.

Step 7. It's 4:00 p.m. Guess who is at the gate? The agent who sent us to United. She looks at us and says that we need to wait until she gets the flight at the gate out of the gate area. Then she does a double take. "Aren't you the ones I sent to another airline?" Yep. That's us. We tell her that there weren't any seats for us. She promises to pursue it with her supervisor and asks if we would like to spend the night in Vegas or DFW since there is no way we will make it home to Iowa that day. One of our disgruntled passengers lays her head on the counter and pouts. There are heavy sighs coming from her.

We are booked on the 6:00 p.m. flight to DFW and told we will get a room voucher for a hotel from the gate agent when we arrive. She hands us a thirty-six-dollar food voucher for our inconvenience. I just laugh. Gene calls and starts rescheduling his patients for the next day. The cancer clinic is closed, so I will have to call in the morning. The Disgruntled One is busy texting her displeasure to the world.

Step 8. We board our plane to Dallas and sigh in relief. Not so fast! I notice the pilot talking to a stewardess, and she is pointing to another passenger. Oh boy. The pilot walks to a seat a few rows behind us and has a discussion with a passenger. He then walks to the front of the plane and makes an announcement: "Ladies and gentlemen. I apologize for the delay, but we have a passenger experiencing medical issues, and we are waiting for the paramedics." Thirty minutes later, the paramedics have wheeled the passenger from the plane. Announcement 2: "We thank you for your patience. But now we are without a ground crew, and it will be a few minutes before we can get a push back from the gate." Super. The Disgruntled One is slumping in her seat.

Step 9. We land at DFW at 11:00 p.m. No restaurants are open in the airport, so the voucher does us no good. The gate agent is very helpful and hands us vouchers for two discounted rooms at a nearby hotel: sixty-nine dollars for each room. We don't care. We need sleep. She calls the hotel and tells us to go out to the baggage claim and walk outside and wait for the shuttle. Things are looking up: a free shuttle! We wait and wait and wait. Gene finds an American employee, who says, "You need to go downstairs to find the hotel shuttles." Super. We go downstairs, and there is no one there. It is now 11:40 p.m. We decide to call the hotel on the shuttle phone, but the number has been disconnected. We decide to get a cab. There are no more cabs because the last flight for the day came in about forty minutes ago. Gene finds another employee, who calls a cab for us.

Step 10. The cabbie asks which hotel we are going to, north or south. We don't know. We show him the address. I figure this isn't going to end well. He tells us there is a $27.50 minimum for any ride out of the airport. We don't care at this point. He drives us to the south hotel location, and we are at the correct hotel. Someone traveling with us is surly to the hotel clerk. Someone needs her nap. Gene and I are exhausted and kiss the beds in our room, but we are too wired up to sleep.

Day 2. Step 11. Back at the airport at 6:30 a.m. after a refreshing four hours of sleep. I get a pat-down by the TSA. I'm still extremely sore, and my skin is oozing from radiation. I ask the agent to be *very* careful. She is. We sit at the gate, and I stare at my thirty-six-dollar food credit. It seems like such a waste not to use it. I tell Gene that I'm going to Starbucks to get us coffee.

The girl at the counter says that they can accept the voucher, but she can't give me change back. She suggests I stock up. Danielle and I buy every granola bar in their counter, three cups of coffee, a package of almonds, a package of pretzels, and three brownies. The total: $35.40. Bingo! I'm happy. I take my grocery sack back to the gate and grin from ear to ear. Gene laughs. My phone rings. Our flight is delayed. I just laugh and tell Gene we better not tell the Disgruntled One. She is scary.

We wait until she asks why we aren't boarding. The disappointment she experiences from being delayed once again requires her to send multiple text messages. I call the cancer center and schedule my chemo for later in the day. I tell them if I don't show up, start without me!

Step 12. We land in Cedar Rapids in a violent storm. We taxi to within sight of the terminal, and we hear the pilot (I kid you not) say, "Unfortunately, the ground crew is not allowed to work when there is lightening in the vicinity, so we will park over here until the storm passes." Someone in our party groans. I snicker. All I have to look forward to is chemo, so I don't care.

Step 13. Fifteen minutes later, we are allowed to proceed to the terminal and exit the plane. We are all making bets about our luggage at this point. We go to the lost luggage counter and explain what happened. The agent asks how many bags we have, and we say three. He looks hesitant and says, "Let's go see what we have." Oh heck. Is it a bad thing to pray that if there is a lost bag, it be mine? Thankfully, we find all three bags. Two have flown

United. One has flown American. All arrived the night before.

That is how it takes thirty-six hours to travel from Vegas to Iowa. When people ask what happened, I reply, "Everything." I received multiple congratulations when I showed up at chemo, but I was the last patient to leave the building. I got to meet the cleaning crew.

After I sent the letter to the airline, they sent me a travel voucher for the full amount of our trip. While the trip from hell may not have been a good reflection on them, they certainly offered great customer support in trying to make up for it.

Sisters

Thursday, June 27: My sister sent me the following e-mail today:

Subject: Your Horoscope today
Your ability to connect with others is quite strong today, so reach out to that estranged family member or new cutie in your life. It's a great time to show that you really understand them deeply.
I found this interesting. You are always able to connect with others.
Love,
Tammy

Here is my reply to her:

Well then, along that line, I have to tell you about a special moment in Vegas. I have avoided looking into the mirror since I lost my hair seven months ago. It only got worse when I lost my eyelashes and eyebrows. I would look at the reflection and feel confusion. Who was that person? She looked familiar, but I didn't know her. She didn't reflect the strength and courage that I felt. It was amazing how easy it was to avoid her eyes. I wasn't embarrassed by my reflection, just confused.

I was looking forward to getting my makeup done for the wedding because I knew there was a possibility that I would have eyelashes and eyebrows, even if only for a day. Just a few moments to remember normalcy. The makeup artist seemed to work for hours layering one thing after another on my face. She asked my preferences and dislikes. I just kept responding, "Ask Danielle." Danielle has always done my makeup for special occasions. She does it much better than I do. Finally, the makeup artist finished and asked if I was ready to see myself.

When I looked into the mirror, I was shocked. I saw you, Tammy. You have always been so much better than me at applying makeup. I have envied you that ability. When I saw my reflection, I cried. Not only did I look normal, I looked better than normal. I looked the best I could…like a reflection of you. The makeup artist patted my shoulder and whispered softly as she dried the tears.

I love you, sister.

Driving Solo

Saturday, July 13: I took my first solo trip this week. I had a medical foundation board meeting in Des Moines, so I packed my bag and my briefcase and took off on a road trip. I was dressed in business attire and wearing makeup, my shoes were slipped off, and I had my tunes turned up and an iced tea in the cup holder. It felt so normal. But I could tell that Gene was worried. "Do you have a full tank of gas? Be sure to stop if you get tired," he said. With a wave, a big grin on my face, and a promise to call when I arrived, I took off on the two-and-a-half-hour drive. I felt like such a big girl!

I used to travel by myself all over the country for meetings and speaking engagements, and I have made the trip to Des Moines or Chicago too many times to count. But I haven't been anywhere farther than Cedar Rapids (thirty miles) unescorted or without a "handler" since last September. I had forgotten how creative I can be on a long drive with music cranked up. Opportunities to expand the foundation and good stories to post on my blog filled my brain. I even spent some time thinking about what I want to do in the next chapter in my life. I'm ready for a challenge.

As I drove into Des Moines, I realized how long it had been since I had driven in heavy traffic. The man behind me tailgated me as I followed the speed limit. I could tell he was getting frustrated (note, I was going the speed limit, and I was in the right-hand lane), and as he passed me, I was prepared to get flipped off. As he got beside me, I could see him scowl and raise his hand to flip me off, when he noticed my nearly bald head and lowered his arm. I bit my lip in order not to laugh until after he passed me. What am I going to do for entertainment once I have more hair?

I noted the changes in the landscape as I drove to the medical society building. When I pulled up, I was hit with the memory of my last visit to the office. It was the day I was diagnosed with cancer. Tess met me in the parking lot that day, and we sat in her car as she cried. How far I have come since September. And what a long journey it has been.

Gene and I felt it was probably too much for me to try to drive home after my meeting, so I drove to Tess's house to spend the night. Tess lives in a small town, like I do, that is no bigger than a mustard stain on a map. We both tease each other about which town will be the first to grow to a point that it is entitled to bold type on the map. So when I got to Polk City and nothing looked familiar, I was a bit concerned. I didn't realize they had a grocery store now. (She wins!) But I decided that I couldn't possibly get lost, so I just kept driving until something looked familiar and I knew where I was. Gene was on the phone with me at the time, and I could picture him holding his head in his hands as I wandered through the streets. "I've got it," I told him. Then, "Oh shoot. I just passed Tess's driveway."

After a night filled with laughter, I drove home without incident the next morning…just in time to get my chemo bag ready for treatment day. Bummer!

What's Next?

Wednesday, July 24: Do you think doctors lie awake at night and come up with tests to run on their patients? I do. I'm pretty sure that when my doctors get bored, they think up some test to put me through just to see what I will say about it. There seems to be an endless supply of tests that we can run to tell me I'm doing just fine. I met with my doctor last week, and we talked about "What's next?"

I'm at a stage where I should begin antihormone medications. Most people have heard about tamoxifen on the news. It is a pill that breast cancer survivors take for five years to help prevent recurrence. Well, it turns out tamoxifen is for premenopausal women, and because I had a birthday, I'm now considered postmenopausal. Who knew? It is like a line in the sand. You are on one side of it or the other. I was just happy to make it to my birthday! Then I find out I'm not only a year older but have also moved to the "post" category. I'm fine with it because there are fewer serious side effects for Arimidex. Unfortunately, there are some significant side effects.

The main side effects with Arimidex are bone loss and an increase in cholesterol. So my oncologist told me that I would need a bone density scan to use as a baseline as well as a cholesterol check. These are easy tests and you don't even have to study for them, but I probably should have studied, because I failed the cholesterol test. Bummer! Do you think I shouldn't have had a hamburger for dinner the night before? The net result of adding Arimidex to my prescription list was that I now have to take six cholesterol pills and two calcium pills a day. So that takes my daily pill count up to fourteen pills a day. I need a pill secretary. Gene says I am going to need a separate bag for my medications when we travel. Funny guy! Wait till he finds out I scheduled him for a colonoscopy!

Once I get through with these tests, I will get to meet with my surgeon to talk about "What's next?" from a surgical standpoint. Funny, isn't it?

Adapting

Tuesday, July 30: My doctors have told me repeatedly to wear sunscreen when I'm outside. What they don't know is that I have been a dedicated sunscreen user since I turned forty and had to have a skin cancer removed from my lower lip. When doctors start cutting pieces off of you, you don't need encouragement to use sunscreen. You just do it. So it has been interesting to play with my doctors by using tanning lotion to get a "fake bake." One of my favorite treatment days was when both my radiologist and my oncologist took a look at my tanned arms and legs and gave me the sunscreen lecture. When I told them that it was tanning lotion, they were surprised. I gave myself a high five and grinned from ear to ear!

Now that my radiation site has healed and I'm feeling better, I'm doing my share of the mowing again. It takes us two-and-a-half hours to mow using two commercial riding lawn mowers. I have yet to find a sunscreen that will hold up that long, so I do get a bit of a tan on my arms. I refuse—refuse, I tell you—to wear long sleeves on a hot, humid day. (Gene does this, and I want to give him full credit for it.) So when I started mowing again, I knew I needed to protect my head, face, and neck beyond sunscreen. My solution was to buy a hat that guarantees SPF 50 or above from a company that specializes in attire for skin cancer patients. The hat has stylish flaps that cover your ears and neck. It is lightweight and cool to wear. Granted, you look ridiculous and like you are about to go on a safari, but you are covered and protected. I did find that my noise-canceling headphones will work with the hat if I turn the volume up a bit. Add a pair of sunglasses and I'm stylin'! I don't worry about what the neighbors will think, because they need binoculars to even see us in the yard.

Finding My Voice

Thursday, August 15: I'm not really sure when I stopped singing, but Gene mentioned the other day, "You are singing again." I think it was more of an observation than a complaint, but you never know. I also think it is a sign that my life is returning to normal. When I'm happy, I tend to sing and not realize it. I crank the music up and sing along, though the words don't always match the lyrics. I always worry when I'm on an airplane that I will forget where I am, and a stewardess will have to come tap me on the shoulder to tell me I'm bothering the other passengers. I'm not a particularly good vocalist, but I put a lot of heart into it.

I have also returned to working regularly. I was particularly lucky that we weren't dependent on my income, so I didn't have to work during treatment. Now that I'm feeling better, I find I need that creative outlet to keep my brain occupied and to keep me out of trouble. My son took over my business for me while I was undergoing treatment and has done a wonderful job of taking care of my clients and helping to grow the business. I think there will be room for both of us to keep busy as we expand.

In an effort to stay current with new technology, I signed up for an online software class recently, and I find that the chemo has altered my ability to absorb new information. I still struggle to remember words, names, and facts. But I'm getting better all the time. The class is a challenge, and it takes me longer to do a lesson than in the past, but I refuse to let computer software stump me, so I plow on through the lessons. On the bright side, with my memory loss, I have lots of books that I have read that I can read over again and they will be new to me. It makes me laugh when I think about it that way.

I have also resumed my love/hate relationship with my long driveway. On good days, I call it the mile-long drive. Other days, I call it torture. My driveway offers half a mile of beautiful, peaceful scenery overlooking the Cedar River. The walk down is great, but the return trip is all uphill. And it isn't a small hill. Since we have lived here, I have walked the drive twice daily with my companions, Gene and Dolly Dog. During treatment, I had to give up the long climb because I was too weak to make it uphill that far. Now the walk is part of my morning routine. I have a lot to sing about.

Minor Inconvenience

Friday, August 23: I was on the phone with someone yesterday trying to schedule a time for a service man to come to my house. When asked what day worked best for me, I replied, "Any day but Thursday. I have chemo that day." The lady on the phone immediately changed her voice to a soft, sympathetic tone. I then said, "Oh, no worries. It is just a minor inconvenience." Seriously? When did I decide that chemo was a minor inconvenience? I had to laugh when I got off the phone, and I'm pretty sure I told Gene yesterday morning that I was annoyed about having to go to chemo.

Maybe cancer has stages like the stages of grief. At first you walk around waiting for someone to tell you there has been a mistake and you really don't have cancer. That is followed by your life being turned upside down and your orderly schedule being tossed out and replaced by dozens of doctor's visits, tests, and labs. That is followed by a mountain of paperwork, forms, and insurance claims. Each time you have to say "I have cancer" out loud, your heart races. Then you start treatment, and you focus on living from one chemo infusion to the next or on getting through radiation. You don't look to the future; you look to the end of treatment. And then you start getting your life back, and you consider infusions (treatment) to be a minor inconvenience.

This is an interesting stage for me. I feel good. I don't take naps as often. I have most of my old energy level back...and I really don't want to spend any more time getting infusions. Like I told the nurse yesterday, "I feel good, and I'm wondering what I'm doing here." She gets it. No lectures on "We are doing everything we can to..." She simply acknowledges that I'm getting better and want to be outside playing rather than hooked to an IV and stuck in a very nice, comfortable chair.

I ran down the stairs to Gene's office yesterday morning, stopped at the bottom, and gave myself a high five. I had just run down a flight of stairs. Like the old days—before chemo.

Unsupervised

Friday, August 23: I had my first unsupervised chemo visit yesterday. Up until now, each time I went to chemo, treatment was preceded by labs and a doctor's visit. But now that I'm doing so well and just having maintenance infusions, I have to see the doctor only every other visit. So this was my first visit without seeing the doctor. I feel like such a big girl.

I was hoping to avoid the dreaded scale on this visit as well, but no such luck. They weigh you so often during treatment that they make Weight Watchers clients look like slackers. On days where I had radiation and chemo on the same day, I got weighed in both visits. You know I couldn't let this go without comment. The first time, I asked what happened to their fancy new electronic medical records. Couldn't the computer on the first floor talk to the computer on the third floor? Hmm? The second time I got weighed twice, I asked the first nurse to write my weight on a piece of paper and sign and date it. I then handed it to the second nurse, and she laughed. The least they could do is have the scale play applause when you lose weight.

My favorite scheduler congratulated me on having only an infusion scheduled and no doctor's appointment. Then she went and jinxed it by saying, "So you are only here for half an hour today?" I cringed. Sure enough, two hours later I walked out of the building. Gene says they keep me that long because I'm so darn entertaining and they get to see me only every three weeks.

Insurance

Friday, August 30: One of the annoyances of having cancer is that you have to deal with insurance constantly. With a fifteen-month treatment plan, I get so much communication with my insurance company that I could get lost in the paperwork. I can't imagine how I would have handled this during the rough stages of chemo and radiation without help. Fortunately, I have a secret weapon—Gene. When family members complain that they don't understand their insurance and insurance choices, Gene replies, "No one does." I beg to differ. Gene has set up a database to track my health-care charges and payments, and he keeps on top of it. He is Superman!

Every couple of months, Gene will stick his head out of his office and ask, "What did you have done on July thirty-first?" Heck if I know. But my calendar is the master plan of my life, so I consult it and tell him what treatment or test I had done. He then explains why the charge is being denied, and we usually have a good laugh. Here are some examples:

In July, a charge for $465 was denied because it appeared that it was a cosmetic procedure, which my insurance would not cover. I checked my calendar, and this was a follow-up radiation appointment. Let me tell you: if I'm going to have cosmetic surgery, it won't be done in radiation!

Another charge resulted in a letter from the insurance company that the charge appeared to be for a work-related injury and I should file it through my employer's workers' comp insurance. My calendar swears that I had gone in for a heart scan to make sure the chemo wasn't damaging my heart too much. I don't know what kind of work these people think I do, but I'm self-employed, I don't have workers' comp insurance, *and* I build websites. Hmm.

Most of the other issues were coding errors and easily fixed once we contacted the hospital or physician's office or insurance company, but a person has to stay on top of their charges or have Superman on their team. A good master calendar doesn't hurt either. Thank you, Gene!

One Year

Tuesday, September 10: Last week marked one year since I started my journey with breast cancer. Though I didn't know it at the time, that morning a year ago would mark the last of my quiet morning routines for some time. Gene and I got up and enjoyed our usual morning walk with Dolly on a crisp September morning. I remember turning to Gene at one point and saying, "I love this time of year," and he grinned and said, "I know you do." Later that morning, I found the lump in my breast as I showered, and the next morning, my father died.

I look back now at that person I was, the things I worried about or stressed over, my priorities, and my goals and find that some things are the same, but so many things are different. I always felt I was a strong person, but I have found strength that I did not know I had. I have always hated to ask for help or rely on others, but I have found peace in asking for help and leaning on a friend or family member when I need to. I have learned so many things about myself, and I suspect that I have changed some attitudes and habits for life.

Gene and I took this week to travel to Texas and be with our family. It was both a joyful weekend as we had a family wedding reception for our son and new daughter as well as a difficult week as we recognized the one-year anniversary of my father's death. Mom and I talked about our two respective mornings of finding the lump and then Dad's death. We are both haunted by those mornings but learning to find some peace. I found myself wondering why we put so much importance on the anniversary of someone's death, but I believe it is part of the healing process. I do know that I'm glad we went home to be with family.

The one-year mark brings another reminder—time for my mammogram! Can you believe it? I should be able to finish treatment before I'm due for that test, don't you think? It is kind of like owning a new car. In my mind, you should have it paid off before you have to replace the tires. (My husband always laughs when I make this comment.)

As you can imagine, I am facing this mammogram in my usual style—with humor. When I called to make my appointment, I asked the scheduler to put a note in my chart that I want them to get it right this year. "No surprises," I say. I want a nice, normal mammogram. Because I live in a small town and have my mammogram at the local hospital, I actually have the e-mail address of the girls in the X-ray department. So I e-mailed them to ask if I get a discount on my mammogram since I have only one breast. Seriously, I did e-mail them. Their response? "We hope your mammogram is uneventful this year! And you do get a discount!" I gave myself a high five. I do love a discount. I will let you know what other trouble I can find when I'm there next month.

Finally, I want to say that I could not, could not have survived this year without the support of Team Kathy. The food, the phone calls, the hugs, the e-mails, the cards, the rides to and from chemo, the company at chemo, the prayers, all the pink gifts, and yes, even the knitting and painting lessons showed me that you cared and were sharing my journey. God blessed me with the angels I needed to help hold me up this past year. I will hold each of you in my heart and prayers forever.

Hot Flashes

Wednesday, September 18: Gene and I were talking about hot flashes tonight, and I laughed until my sides hurt. When I was in phase one of chemo, I was given steroids to counteract some side effects of chemotherapy. What the doctors don't tell you is that you have side effects from the steroids they prescribe to minimize other side effects. In the past, I have avoided taking steroids because they make me mean and hungry. Not necessarily in that order. The steroids for chemo may be a bit different, because they caused hot flashes and the inability to sleep.

My kids laugh at the story about my first hot flash. I woke up at two in the morning burning up. I was certain that the heat between my neck and my pillow would cause me to spontaneously combust. I remember jumping out of bed, putting my hands on my hips, and stating (loudly), "I'm hot!" Gene, being the good sport that he is, mumbled, "Okay." That wasn't good enough for me. I glared at him and then marched in and pressed the down button on the thermostat until I felt it was sufficient and returned to bed.

A couple of hours later, I woke to find myself bundled under the covers with just my cold nose poking out. I turn to see Gene mummified as well. When I checked the thermostat the next morning, it read sixty degrees. There may have been frost on the inside of the windows. Gene's comment: "Well, at least the air conditioning is working." It was December in Iowa.

The hot flashes went away after I no longer needed the steroids, but they have come back with the inclusion of Arimidex in my prescription lineup. Arimidex (similar to tamoxifen) is prescribed to help prevent cancer from returning. I have been fortunate not to have any menopausal symptoms up until this point, but within two weeks of taking Arimidex, I began to have hot flashes. When my doctor asked me about hot flashes, I said, "Yes, and I want to thank you for that." She appreciates my humor.

So, to all my friends who have complained about hot flashes over the years—I'm sorry. I was not nearly as sympathetic as I should have been.

Going Pink for October

Tuesday, October 1: Well, it is official. I have gone pink for Breast Cancer Awareness Month! Shawn dyed a section of my hair pink over the weekend, so I won't have to worry about wearing pink all month. Dying my hair was quite the experience. If you know me well, I dress conservatively (normally) and try not to stand out in a crowd. So dying my hair was a huge leap for me. I was so nervous as Shawn showed me the colors to pick from, and I found myself coming up with excuses for why I should reconsider. But then I made the statement, "If I don't do it now, I will never do it." So Shawn strapped me in, and away we went. I remember telling him that I wanted subtle (pink?) and not to look like a clown. "You know how a clown has big poufy hair in a bunch of different colors?" Shawn just laughed and said, "You don't have big poufy hair to start with." Good to keep the humor flowing. I will tell you that Gene is a patient man. He sat in the chair and graciously waited as Shawn stripped my hair of color and then dyed it pink. Not once, but twice. We think that due to the number of medications in my system, my hair did not want to go pink for October. It is stubborn like me.

Not only have I gone pink for October, but I'm having my mammogram done today. I ask each of you to do a self-exam and schedule your mammogram if it is due. I found my lump myself, and science shows that early detection improves your chance of survival.

Mammogram (Not!)

Wednesday, October 2: Several weeks ago, I got an e-mail reminder that my mammogram was due. Really? Shouldn't I be allowed to finish treatment for breast cancer before I have to do another mammogram? But I was a good sport and went ahead and scheduled my mammogram for October 1. Why not get it done in Breast Cancer Awareness Month?

As the date approached, I found myself getting more and more nervous about the test. My oncologist told me that she would be shocked if anything was spotted on my X-rays. She said that they have pumped me so full of chemo meds the past year that she cannot imagine a cancer cell getting by. Gene said basically the same thing, but the mind is a funny thing. And my mind says I won't be comfortable until this is behind me.

My plan (which was a good plan) was to go to my local hospital and have the test done, then walk upstairs and take Gene to lunch. Might as well have some fun with it, right? When I walk into radiation, I announce that I want "a good technician who will get my test right." They laugh. They are expecting me. My tech says, "Sure. No pressure!" Things go as expected, and I'm asked to disrobe and come into the mammogram room. When I go to remove my top, I see a basket of breast cancer awareness goodies (hand sanitizer, nail files, mints, pens) and a stack of "Laugh with Kathy" business cards referring people to my blog. Aww! How fun is this? And I happen to need a nail file.

I enter the mammogram room and it hits me—this is where it all started, in this darn room. I really, really don't want to be here. But then, I really don't want to have cancer again, so knowing is better than not knowing. We squish my breast in the machine, and the tech takes the first photo—and I hear the tech groan. This can't be good. She assures me that we were lined up well and the image is good, except something is wrong with the machine and it isn't developing or loading correctly. She tells me this has happened before and asks for a few minutes to try to get the machine to cooperate. The machine does not cooperate. The machine does not know it is Breast Cancer Awareness Month and that I really, really need it to give me a normal mammogram.

A second tech comes in to look at the machine, and I think they are about to call a code blue on it. I'm wondering if we can shock it with one of those wall-mounted defibrillators. That would be fun, and it would serve it right. Nope, they can't fix it, and there is no way a radiologist is going to be able to read my X-ray. They explain that they are closed for the next three days for a system upgrade, so I will need to come back in a week or so. Seriously? I can't make this stuff up.

I go back to Gene's office, and he looks up expectantly. "How did it go?" he asks. "I broke the machine," I respond. He just holds his head. Now is when he gets to tell me that he has to do an emergency surgery and can't go to lunch with me. My great plan just went down the toilet. And I'm not even going to get a good lunch out of it! Is it too early for a drink? Do you think I'm being penalized for only having one breast and asking for a discount?

I call Tess on the way home, and she starts laughing and says, "You know what the problem is? God just wants to give you more material for your blog!"

Race for the Cure

Wednesday, October 16: Over the past year, many of you have walked in your local Race for the Cure and sent me photos or told me that you were walking for me. It would be impossible to tell you how much this simple act means to someone going through breast cancer treatment. As the time approached for our local walk, I debated whether or not I should attend. In the end, I told Gene that I wasn't ready yet. His reply: "That's okay. We can do our own walk." The perfect response as always.

One of the reasons I don't want to do the walk yet is because I don't feel like a survivor. I haven't finished treatment, so in my mind, I'm still a patient. I have talked with other survivors and my doctors, who tell me that I can call myself a survivor whenever I want to. One person told me that you become a survivor the day you learn of your diagnosis and decide to fight to live. I get their point, but I won't use that word until I'm done with treatment in January.

The other reason I don't want to participate in a walk is because I think I will cry. Each time I get an e-mail or photo from a friend or relative who tells me they walked for me, I cry. I can't help it. I cry because I'm deeply touched. I cry because I want to be the person walking for someone else. I cry for all the breast cancer patients who didn't survive. When I see a sea of people walking wearing pink T-shirts with photos on their sleeves, I cry.

We happened to be in town this weekend when the Race for the Cure participants had finished their walk and streamed into a local restaurant for coffee and breakfast. I felt the tightness in my chest and the tears near the surface. I saw angel wings and a person's name on a sleeve. As soon as I got outside, I started gulping in breaths of fresh air and trying to hold on until we got into the car. Tears streamed down my face, and Gene quietly drove us home. He waited until I felt I could talk and express my thoughts. He is a kind and considerate man.

I told him that every time my nieces walk and wear my photo next to their Aunt Rhonda's photo, my heart breaks. Why is it that I am surviving my battle with cancer, when she lost her battle? I pray that I can help others who are struggling with cancer or have a family member struggling with cancer understand the journey, or at least let them know that it is okay to cry and laugh along the way. I may never be able to actively participate in a Race for the Cure, but I respect and appreciate those who do.

The Big Gamble

Friday, November 1: It had been a long time since one of my friends called and asked me to blow off whatever plans I had and take a day to play. So when Tess called and suggested we meet for lunch, I was all in. Meeting Tess for lunch involves an hour's drive for each of us since we live two hours apart. And the only thing in the middle of rural Iowa is a casino. So could we help it if we found ourselves at a casino on Tuesday? I have so missed getting into trouble!

Once we decided to shirk our duties of work and volunteerism, we put on our oldest clothing and drove to our meeting point. We elect to wear old clothing because the smoke in the casino permeates our clothes to the point it has to be burned or washed several times to get the smell out. Coats and jackets were removed and left in the car as we dashed inside, laughing the entire way.

The great thing about going to a casino during the middle of the week is that it makes you feel young. Busloads of retirees are dropped off just before lunch and depart again around half past two. So two laughing "less than retirees" tend to stand out. And the fact that we have no idea how to gamble makes us stand out even more. But I have found that if you feed the machine money and press a button, something will happen. We clap and squeal as we win $1.20, and the people gambling next to us get up and leave. This makes us laugh harder. The security guard walks up behind us and says, "You girls seem to be having fun!" (Did someone call security on us?) No alcohol is served at this casino, so we are laughing simply for the joy of living.

We have just about exhausted our time when I tell Tess about my research money. I participate in a clinical trial for cancer patients as a way to "pay it forward" to future cancer patients. I feel deeply indebted to previous patients who did trials that have helped me in my treatment. As part of the trial, I am paid ten dollars a month to participate. When I tried to decline the payment, I was told that the paperwork to do that was daunting and it was better if I just took the money and used it for something fun. So I checked my clinical debit card, and I had twenty dollars to spend. I told Tess that we needed to find a fun machine and blow my fortune.

We searched for the perfect machine and found a pretty, shiny one to put my money into. We were down to about two dollars when I hit the free-spin bonus. The machine kept spinning and spinning, and we kept laughing and laughing. Lights were going off as we laughed until our sides hurt. People stopped to stand behind us, and we held our sides and laughed at each spin. I'm not going to go into details, but the amount I won (while not enough to fund the research study) was noteworthy—at least to two amateur gamblers. I couldn't hit the payout button fast enough. Needless to say, we are not the gamblers the casino is looking for.

The Friend

Friday, November 8: I have a friend who will be going through chemo with me, and I feel sorry for him. It turns out that not every type of chemo causes you to lose your hair. His particular chemotherapy has its own set of side effects, but he will get to keep his hair. I find this sad. He won't get to experience all the perks that come with being bald:

- He won't get seventeen hats for Christmas.
- He won't get to make people feel bad for cutting him off when he is driving.
- He won't get the extra-large portions or get served first at restaurants.
- People won't offer to let him cut in line or take their seat in a waiting room.
- He won't be able to wash and dry his head in under thirty seconds.
- He won't save any money on hair products and haircuts.
- He can't doze off in a boring meeting and get away with it.

I want to make it up to him, so we have scheduled our chemo for the same time next week. We plan to raise hell at the cancer clinic and get away with it. After all, we are poor cancer patients.

Put Me on the Cancer Bus!

Friday, December 6: As I am checking in for my appointments at the cancer clinic, the receptionist slides a flier over to me and tells me that she wants to let me know about the special holiday plans for cancer patients. My humor radar goes into overdrive as I glance at the list of activities.

The first thing the receptionist tells me about is the annual wreath competition and giveaway. Patients are encouraged to view the wreaths on display and vote for their favorite. A patient's name is drawn for each wreath, and the patient gets to keep the wreath. This is all new and exciting to the receptionist, who started work at the clinic after the holidays last year. I tell her that I have been there for *all* the holidays in 2013, so if she has any questions, just ask. She laughs and says, "They should put you on the committee!"

Next on the list of exciting events for cancer patients is the Christmas party at the cancer clinic. I tell her, "Oh, that is exactly where I want to spend my Christmas." By now, both receptionists are laughing. As I look through the list of activities for the Christmas cancer party, I see that they are chartering a bus to take the patients and their family members to look at Christmas lights. I can just see it now: "Come on, kids. Let's get on the cancer bus and go look at Christmas lights!" I laugh as I go sit down and wait for my turn for labs. I'm so glad they get my sense of humor.

Acts of Kindness

Monday, December 30: One of the things that have touched me beyond words has been the incredible acts of kindness that people have shown me during my treatment. Some were from family members or good friends; others were from casual acquaintances. I couldn't begin to list them all, but a simple card in the mail today reminded me of the generosity and compassion of others.

A friend of mine mailed me a note card that she has had in her desk for the past ten years. The cover is an image of a quilt that a woman made to depict the diagnosis, treatment, and coping a woman goes through in her journey with breast cancer. The card itself would have been a considerate gesture, but the fact that she held on to it for ten years in order to find the right person to send it to, and that she chose me, touches me.

Almost as soon as I was diagnosed, people started sending me things. I think it is a way of "doing something" when you don't know what else to do. At times, I couldn't deal with these gifts. Either I was too overwhelmed with the gesture, too tired, or too sick, but I had the forethought to put a container in my office to hold all the items. I recently went through the basket and found some surprises. I found a lucky rock that my friend sent me. Her note says that she found the rock when she was ten years old and it has always brought her luck. How touching that someone would share something they have held dear for nearly forty years. I plan to return the rock to her as soon as I'm done with treatment.

I found a crossword puzzle book that I have started working on to help with the chemo brain. I have trouble remembering words, and some days I will work on a clue for days and then jump for joy when I finally remember the word. So far, I have resisted the use of Google to help complete the puzzles, and Gene laughs when I tell him that I'm tempted to ask the nurses for help on a science or medical clue. But each time I get closer to completing a puzzle, I find a sense of accomplishment. Unfortunately, I can't remember who gave me the puzzle book! Ironic, isn't it?

Some gifts were very practical and were used immediately. My chemo bag has a prayer blanket to keep me warm at chemo, a pair of warm and soft pink socks, the most beautiful shawl (which made me the envy of all other chemo patients), ChapStick, a Dammit Doll (in case it is one of those frustrating days), cheese crackers and a granola bar (in case of famine), a pen and paper, and my Kindle loaded with books friends have shared.

Some gifts were funny—a bracelet with a pair of testicles that reads "It takes balls to beat cancer!," a bra purse, a chemo fairy, bubble gum and coloring books (for those who know I get bored easily), and so many more. Some gifts were touching—the personal notes of encouragement that seemed to arrive when I needed them most, the text message from my sister-in-law on the morning of every chemo appointment. And some gifts were the gift of time—the friends and family who sat with me during my chemo appointments and watched over me as I slept.

In the end, the actual gift didn't matter. All of these things remind me that I matter and that I am cared for. I know I have a tremendous team of people who are supporting me through this journey. I hope that this experience makes me a better friend and that my words and sharing my experience help someone else through their journey.

Early Celebration

Wednesday, January 1, 2014: After exhausting the Iowa pumpkin supply, Gene and I traveled to Texas over the holidays to celebrate the near end of my treatment with my family. Gene has marked the completion of each chemo session these past fifteen months by blowing up a pumpkin or watermelon for me. With only one infusion left in my treatment, we wanted to have an early celebration with my family.

I asked my family members to come "dressed to kill," which has a special meaning in Texas. Each family member wore various camo-colored shirts, hats, and accessories. Some carried weapons. My mom's weapon of choice was a camo-colored flashlight. I'm not sure what she planned to do with it, but it made me laugh as she clutched it in her hand. Maybe she was the light at the end of the tunnel. As we gathered for a group photo, I looked around and thought about the support that they have given me this past year. So many e-mails and cards and text messages. Their messages of support and caring gave me strength to see my treatment to the end.

Since pumpkins are scarce in Texas as well this time of year, we celebrated by blowing up melons, piñatas, and water jugs. I sat with my mother as my brother-in-law took the first shot and exploded the piñata. Mom's eyes were huge, and I laughed as confetti flew in every direction. It doesn't get better than that. The neighbor's horses and dog barely even flinched at the noise. You could tell we were in Texas! There is something cathartic about watching things blow up. One minute they are there, and the next minute they are in a hundred pieces. Next came the water jugs, and most everyone took a turn at a target. I was impressed that everyone hit their target on the first try. They must have been practicing.

After the water jugs and piñata were killed, it was time to shoot some melons. When I asked everyone to bring their own targets, I suggested something organic. I used the excuse that the birds and animals would then clean up the mess, and we wouldn't leave a lot of debris in Mom's field. In reality, I made the suggestion because there is something funny about watching food explode. I was entertained with stories from my family about trips to the Asian and Hispanic food markets in search of the perfect fruit to blow up.

I have to admire the women in this family because they are excellent shots as well. I can hit a target, but I don't care for shooting guns. It is entertaining to watch others shoot though.

We finished our celebration by splitting into several groups and playing cards and dominos. Prizes were available for the best players, and my brother and I won all three rounds of games. My brother suggested we skip out and hit the casino with the luck we were having. I will admit, I was tempted. Spending time with family is so much fun. I will remember this Christmas for the rest of my life.

The Caregiver

Saturday, January 3: Over the past year, I have often wondered whether cancer is worse for the patient or the caregiver. In the first month of diagnosis and treatment, I apologized to Gene no less than two dozen times. He finally turned to me and said, "Knock it off. I would take this burden from you if there was any way possible, but I can't. We are in this together." That stopped me in my tracks. There was no way I would let him or anyone take on my cancer so I could get out of it. I wouldn't wish this on anyone. So we began this journey together, and he has walked each step at my side.

My days were filled with doctor's appointments, procedures, and sometimes simply focusing on living until the next chemo treatment. Gene's days were filled with worry. I watched him and saw the effects of the stress as he tried to make each day easier for me. I saw his strength, his gentleness, his compassion as he asked me to try to eat just two bites of something. He helped me set up a chart for my nausea medications. He walked slowly by my side when I insisted I was going to take a walk and said words of encouragement even when I couldn't walk more than halfway to the shop. And he walked Dolly Dog when I simply couldn't find the strength, and I sat and watched them from the window with tears in my eyes. I saw his frustration when he knew that all he could do was sit by my side. I hated what this disease was doing to him and my children.

But through it all, we found humor. Shortly after I was diagnosed, I decided it was time I taught Gene how to cook so he could survive if I didn't make it through my journey. I remember taking him into the kitchen the week before my mastectomy and saying, "I want to show you how to make a few simple meals."

He said, "No way. You aren't going anywhere." And he turned and walked out of the kitchen. I stood with my mouth open and then laughed. Draw a line in the sand, Gene, and hold to it! We ate a lot of pizza, let me tell you. That man can order a pizza better than anyone.

We had rules about laundry. I would sort the clothes and leave them in piles on the bathroom floor. Gene would carry a pile to the washer, but he wasn't allowed to touch the controls. No way was I going to have both of us wearing pink for the next year. I found a handy dry cleaner who would actually drive to my door and pick up Gene's work clothes and deliver them back the next week. Cool beans!

We laughed so hard at Christmas when the kids opened their gifts, and I was so surprised at what they got even though I was the one who purchased and wrapped them. We would laugh at my memory lapses, and Gene would just shake his head when I watched movies as if it were the first time I had ever seen them. The storage room in the basement was a treasure trove of mystery and entertainment as I would open a box and find new stuff in it.

And I swear it was just for entertainment that Gene purchased me a new vehicle recently. I resisted Gene's and the salesman's attempts to get me to test-drive it. After all, I could barely remember how to drive my current vehicle. At times, I couldn't remember where the cruise control was located or how to operate it. So the learning curve on a new vehicle has been nothing short of hilarious.

The first time I drove it by myself, I had to go to chemo. Just before leaving, Gene called me to tell me that it was raining and asked if I knew how to turn on the windshield wipers. Hmm? No, I have no idea. Gene goes through a five-step process to explain it to me. Seriously? I can't remember three things in a row without writing them down, but I nod on the phone and say, "Got it. Thanks."

Three minutes later, I am in the vehicle, and it turns out it *is* raining. I don't remember anything Gene has told me. I look around and see no source of help. So I sit in the driveway and call him at work. Maybe this will go better if I am actually sitting in the car. He laughs and patiently talks me through what now seems like a seventy-two-step process, offering various alternatives and what-ifs. He can't help it. It is the scientist in him. The wipers appear to be working, and I have no plans on doing anything like making an adjustment until I arrive at my destination. "Got it. Thanks," I say. There is a pause on his end. I can hear the gears in his brain spinning. I grin as I imagine the beads of sweat forming on his brow as he worries about me driving alone. "How hard could it be?" I ask. "Love you," and I hang up.

As my treatment is drawing to an end, I see him relaxing more. He no longer cringes when I drive myself to town. He laughs with me at my forgetfulness and the mistakes I make. Our house is starting to return to normal. We are both ready for life after cancer.

The Finish Line

Saturday, January 18: Years ago, my middle son, Steven, participated in a track meet at his high school and ran the long-distance (five-thousand-meter) event. I sat in the stands with the other parents and watched the race and cheered the runners. As dozens of runners passed him, I watched Steven continue at his own pace, seemingly in his own world. The fastest runners completed the race, followed by most of the other runners, and yet Steven and a few runners continued to run. It was difficult to watch as a parent. I wondered if he felt bad for being near the back of the pack, and my heart ached for him. But slowly, the crowd began to clap and to cheer on the final dozen runners. And Steven started picking up speed. The crowd clapped louder, and he ran faster. He passed one runner after another, and the crowd was roaring as he crossed the finish line. I had tears in my eyes. And Steven? Steven was oblivious. He didn't hear the clapping or notice that he was passing other runners. It turns out that he wasn't running for anyone else but simply for the joy of running. And crossing the finish line was simply the end of the run.

I have carried this memory in my heart for over ten years. Sometimes the finish line is just a moment in the journey. Yesterday was like that for me. It was the thirtieth, and last, infusion for me, but it was just one moment in a long journey.

I had planned my last treatment to fall on a Friday so that Gene could be with me. I wasn't sure how I would feel as I completed treatment. I knew I would be happy to have reached the end, but I wondered if I would also be a bit sad as I said good-bye to my nursing staff.

Gene arrived just as I was being unhooked from my IV, and I was so glad he could share in this moment. Everything is better when he is at my side. The nurses gathered and played "Pomp and Circumstance" on their kazoos and blew bubbles as they rang their bells. It is silly, but it is a celebration. Gene took our picture, and I went and rang the bell loudly. I was doing fine until the nurses each hugged me and whispered words of encouragement. And then tears came to my eyes. Patients and staff were clapping, but I could hardly hear them. How could I possibly thank them for taking care of me and saving my life? In the end, all I could do was whisper, "Thank you." I had reached the finish line.

CHAPTER 7
HAIR GROWTH AND CHEMO BRAIN

In this chapter, I have collected stories about hair growth and chemo brain. While they seem unrelated, they were the two issues that caused me the most grief yet generated some of the most amusing moments. Read along as I deal with missing hair and missing memory.

Almost from the start, I wondered how long it would take me to grow my hair back, what it would look like, and if I would have curls. My doctor told me that my hair would start growing after chemo phase two, but she couldn't tell me how long it would take. So I decided to take photos of my head each week and post them on my blog. I struggled with new hair products and flatirons, and impatience as I waited for my bangs to finally grow.

The first time I heard the phrase "chemo brain" was shortly after I was diagnosed. A breast cancer survivor told me that the best part of having cancer is that you get to claim chemo brain the rest of your life. I don't think the survivor was correct. I think the best part of having cancer is all the new adventures you get to have with chemo brain. Everything is new again: books, movies, people's names, my own phone number. After the initial fear of having lost my memory, I embraced chemo brain and proclaimed, "Every day is an adventure!"

Hair Watch—Week One

Monday, April 8, 2013: Now that I'm done with the chemo that caused my hair to fall out, it is time for me to see how long it takes to grow in. It is week one of waiting for my hair to grow, and there is no sign of hair regrowth. I've got nothin'! I don't care how close you get, there is no hair on my head. But just for grins, I told Gene that I could actually feel my hair growing under the scalp. He laughed. Stay tuned as I chronicle the regrowth of my hair.

Hair Watch—Week Two

Wednesday, April 17: Nope. No sign of hair. However, I used my three-times-magnification makeup mirror and found two stragglers that somehow escaped the lint roller. One is on the top of my head and is about a quarter inch long. The other is above my left ear and is nearly a half inch long. Neither is long enough to curl or use a blow dryer on. I'm almost afraid to touch them in case it causes them to fall out. I am debating on whether or not I should trim them. They seem to have an unfair "head start" on the rest of my hair. I guess I'm going to have to start looking for summer hats. All of my visors leave my scalp uncovered, and I don't want to get sun burned.

Hair Watch—Week Four

Saturday, April 27: Still waiting! Gene tells me that if I stand in the sunlight and he cocks his head just so, he thinks he can see some peach fuzz. I think I can feel a texture change on the scalp. I'm planning to have some fun with the bald head for whatever time I have left with it.

First Haircut

Sunday, April 28: That single hair on the top of my head was getting in my way and threatening to obscure my view. Seriously, it was growing straight up and had no supporting cast to distract from it. I looked through my stylist's hair-product line and found some smoothing paste. But how do you apply it to just one hair? So I had Shawn trim the single hair today. He is the greatest hairstylist of all. He put a cape around my shoulders and checked that single hair from all angles and then snipped it just right. I did tell him on the way out the door that I thought he cut my bangs too short.

Who Moved My Cheese? (Part One)

Monday, October 21: About ten years ago, there was a popular book out titled *Who Moved My Cheese?* that discussed how people react to change. Who knew that ten years later, this phrase would come to mind so often?

One of the side effects of chemo is chemo brain. Doctors and researchers call chemo brain "mild cognitive impairment." Most define it as being unable to remember certain things and having trouble finishing tasks or learning new skills. Here are just a few examples of what patients call chemo brain:

- Forgetting things that they usually have no trouble recalling (memory lapses)
- Having trouble concentrating or focusing on what they're doing, having a short attention span, potential "spacing out"
- Having trouble remembering details like names, dates, and sometimes larger events
- Having trouble multitasking, like answering the phone while cooking, without losing track of one task
- Taking longer to finish things (disorganized, slower thinking and processing)
- Having trouble remembering common words (unable to find the right words to finish a sentence)

I know what many of you are thinking: this happens to everyone at some point. But what you have to understand is that we (cancer patients) have had chemo, so we have a built-in excuse for the rest of our lives. The rest of you are just forgetful!

When I first started noticing chemo brain, it scared me. I couldn't add numbers in my head. I couldn't remember our room number if we were in a hotel. I couldn't remember names of people I have known for years. I would forget words and couldn't finish a sentence. I had difficulty figuring out a menu in my favorite restaurant. My family has been very good to calmly supply the word I'm looking for when I can't seem to come up with it or to order my favorite dishes when I look at a menu in confusion.

I stopped at the bank recently to make a deposit, and the clerk asked if she could help me. I said, "Yes. I don't know the date, and I don't know my account number, but I do know where I am." She laughed and processed my deposit, then pointed south and said, "You live two miles that way." So helpful! But it did make me laugh.

Another example of my confusion was at a charity auction where Gene and I had purchased two items. The cashier read off the cost of the two items that we bought, and I sat with my pen poised over my checkbook, trying to figure out what the total was. I tried to add the two numbers in my head but kept forgetting the first number. I stood helpless until Gene leaned over my shoulder and whispered the total in my ear. I turned and grinned at him and said, "You do realize I'm the treasurer of this fundraiser, don't you?" We both laughed at the irony.

I can't list the number of times I have walked down the hall at home and turned to ask Gene where I'm going or what I was supposed to do. Trying to remember to take my daily medications has resulted in the dreaded pill keeper. Dry-erase boards with lists are my friends. And the list of unfinished tasks is endless.

Chemo brain struck again yesterday when I walked into the grocery store and stopped dead in my tracks. I looked around and thought, "How could they have totally rearranged the store in just three days?" It turns out that I had driven to a different grocery store than I usually go to. Once I realized this, I grinned and nearly clapped my hands. This would be like a scavenger hunt as I tried to find the items I needed! When I got home and told Gene the story, we laughed as we imagined the service desk calling him to tell him they had found me wandering helplessly through the aisles. I told him that the good news is that every day is an adventure and I will never get bored.

One of the best parts of chemo brain is that I don't remember most of the books I have read or the movies I have watched. So I can start over in my wonderful library of books, and they will all be new again. I have moments as I'm reading when things seem a bit familiar or I can guess what is coming next, but then I claim to be psychic. Maybe a day will come when I don't remember that I had cancer...hmm.

Hair Watch—Week Six

Tuesday, May 14: It is official. I have starter hair. Granted, you can't see it without a magnifying glass, but it is there. When I tell my friends that my hair has started to grow, they all do the same thing. They lean in close and inspect my scalp. It makes me laugh.

Hair Watch—Week Ten

Thursday, June 6: Last Friday, I had both chemo and radiation. Everyone asked me what big plans I had for the weekend. My reply was the same: "I'm getting a haircut." They all died laughing. Little did they know that I was serious. Gene was scheduled for his regular haircut with our stylist, and Shawn can't resist a bald head. He shaves his own head, which I think is weird for a hairstylist. In the past, I have always gauged hairstylists' creativity by how they wear their own hair. What does bald say?

When Gene is done with his cut, Shawn puts me in the chair and inspects my head closely. He trims one or two hairs, and then I tell him that this is my wedding haircut. "My son is getting married next week," I tell him.

"No pressure," he says. He looks closely, but it is hard to improve on perfection. Shawn then hands me a box of new hair products that promise to make your hair grow faster and thicker than it is now. I call this a 100 percent certainty considering my head is nearly bald. The box includes shampoo, conditioner, and special drops to put on your scalp afterward.

I ask him, "What happens if I get it on my face?" We laugh.

I now have distinct, dark fuzz all over my head that is less than a quarter inch long. I use one drop of shampoo and feel like I'm drowning in bubbles. I have tiny eyelashes that are too short to use mascara on and a hint of eyebrows. Things are progressing nicely.

Who Moved My Cheese? (Part Two)

Friday, October 25: The last two days have been so funny that I thought I would share my memory lapses with you. Gene and I were watching a home improvement show last night where a couple was pulling up carpet to expose the hardwood flooring underneath. It reminded me of selling our first house twenty-seven years ago. The new owners were going to pull up the carpet after they bought the home and expose the hardwood floors. I have always wondered how that went for them, and then I wondered aloud what that little house would sell for today.

I told Gene that I was going to look it up to see what the current value of that home was. I turned to him and proudly stated, "And I still remember what the street address was."

Gene seemed surprised and asked me, "So what was the address?"

"12345 Thirty-Second Avenue," I told him with a smirk, enjoying my superior memory skills.

He paused and said, "Um, that is our current address."

My face fell. I was so deflated. For a moment there, I felt confident in my superior memory skills, only to find out that I was off by about twenty-seven years. Then I started laughing so hard that my sides hurt. I simply could not catch my breath.

To top it off, for the past two days, Gene and I have been searching the house to find all the cordless phones that seem to have been misplaced. We have a two-story home, and we have five cordless phones placed strategically so that you don't have to run to catch the phone.

Each night, Gene returns the phones to their chargers so that we will remain organized. But for the past two days, he has been searching for all the phones. I'm not sure what happened two days ago that I needed all the phones, but I must have been pretty busy because we could find only two of them. So today, we decided we were going to locate the rest of them one way or another.

Gene asks, "Did you take them outside?"

"No," I reply confidently. Seriously, I don't even remember using all the phones, so one shouldn't put any confidence in my replies. So we search the house, and one by one, we find all of the phones but one. I just can't figure it out. We have searched the house top to bottom—twice. Gene remembers that the phone system has a locator intercom, so he pushes it, and we start following the sound. We look and look until we figure out where the beeps are coming from: my dresser drawer! What could I have possibly been thinking when I put the phone in my dresser? I look at Gene innocently and ask, "Why would you put the phone in there?" We laugh.

I told a friend these stories this morning, and he replied, "Pretty soon you will be able to hide your own Easter eggs!"

Hair Watch—Week Eleven

Thursday, June 13: Ah, week eleven. My brother-in-law and I compared our short hair to see whose was longest. Since he has a short crew cut, I asked him how he decides it is time to trim his hair. He replied, "Whenever I wake up and have bed head." Bed head—something to look forward to!

Hair Watch—Week Fifteen

Tuesday, July 16: I'm done with hats! Seriously. No more stocking caps. No more ball caps. Raquel, the wig, can stay in the drawer. I have hair now, and I'm happy to flaunt it. Granted, it is too short to need styling, but I do use shampoo and conditioner…a drop of each. I tried to borrow my husband's comb this week because the hair on top of my head seems to be growing straight up. I thought maybe I could comb it down. It was too short for Gene's comb, but my eyebrow comb worked very well. I'm finding you have to be creative in problem solving hair issues. I also seem to have this swirl pattern going on. I think I will just wait to see what it does rather than trying to tame it.

The eyebrows are working again. They may be short, but they divert water away from my eyes in the shower. It is amazing to realize that eyebrows and eyelashes actually serve a function and aren't just decorative. I have tried mascara a couple of times, but the lashes are still too short to see a noticeable difference, so mostly I just skip it. And sadly, I'm shaving my legs again. I truly didn't miss this chore.

Directionally Challenged

Wednesday, July 31: About every three months, I have to get a MUGA scan of my heart to make sure the chemo isn't damaging it too much to continue treatments. This is one of those medical tests you don't have to study for and can't screw up because you ate a cheeseburger the night before. The only annoying parts are that you have to have blood drawn (but they give it back to you, unlike other blood tests!), and you have to lie flat on your back for about twenty minutes.

I arrive at the hospital, and I'm determined not to ask for directions to the X-ray department. I have been there three other times for this same test, so surely I can find it on my own…I think. The G (ground) and B (basement) buttons on the elevator confuse me since I'm starting on the ground floor and the side of the elevator says "1," but I cross my fingers and press one of them. In my opinion, as long as I'm going down, I'm bound to be close to my destination. I get off the elevator and nothing looks familiar, but I find some signs that point toward X-ray and pat myself on the back for being close. I giggle as I arrive at X-ray and try not to laugh as I check in. The girls laugh with me when I explain my confusion, and they congratulate me and tell me I'm in the right place.

An X-ray tech comes out to get me and comments that she can see from my chart that I have had this test done before. I reply, "I'm an old hat at this. Just let me know if you have any questions."

She laughs at me, and we approach an intersection in the hallway. She turns left, I turn right. I kid you not! She is laughing and says, "You may know everything there is to know about this test, but you don't know where you are going!" We laugh until our sides hurt. Seriously, movie directors couldn't come up with better timing!

The tech explains the procedure in case I have forgotten anything and quizzes me on things like, "How long do you have to sit and wait after I draw your blood?" She then says she is going to borrow some of my blood but promises to give it back in about twenty-five minutes. I tell her that she is better than the nurses at chemo because they just keep my blood. I sit and wait while she attaches radioactive material to my blood cells before reinjecting them back into me. Then I am told to lie on a table as they begin the test.

I can tell you from experience that laughter and MUGA scans don't mix well. I chuckle a few times thinking about my wrong turn in the hall, and it messes up the test. It is difficult for me to lie still while my brain is going a million miles an hour. I listen to my heartbeat on the speaker, and it increases as I have brilliant ideas and laugh in my head at the outcomes. I'm sure that the tech is writing "noncompliant" on my chart…again.

The tech shows me the images and explains that the left ventricle of my heart looks like a banana and the right looks like an orange or apple. Wait until I freak out the next tech by explaining the image to them. She then sends me on my way and tells me that I have made her day. I tell her she is pretty fun herself and then find my way to my car without incident. Who needs directions?

Hair Watch—Week Seventeen

Tuesday, July 30: When I had the last chemo on March 31, my mom asked me how long it would take for my hair to grow back. I told her that I wouldn't need my first haircut until August. Frankly, I just made that up. I really believed that I would need a cut sooner than that, but it would take until August for it to thicken up. Well, the joke is on me! I still don't need a trim, but I will say that my hair is as thick as it ever was. I'm lucky that way. The swirl pattern continues, and from the back it looks like I walked into a tornado. I suspect that my hair will be curly for a while. I'm okay with that. I have always had heavy, straight, thick hair, so some curl would be an interesting change. I find that getting my hair back isn't as big of a deal as I thought it would be. I have gotten used to being bald.

Hair Watch—Week Nineteen

Tuesday, August 13: My hair continues to grow slowly, and I would estimate that it is about half an inch long now. I find myself a bit surprised by how slowly it is growing—not that I'm complaining. Any hair is better than no hair! I just would have expected it to be longer by now. The hair that I have is very thick, like my old hair, and wavy, not like my old hair. I plan to enjoy whatever comes in and give my stylist free rein over hairstyles for the next year.

One thing I have noticed about this stage in my hair growth is that people look at me differently now. When I was bald, people were very, very nice to me. I tried not to take too much advantage of it, but you have to have a little fun. Now that I have very short hair, people will look at me like they are trying to decide if I'm recovering from cancer or if this is a personal lifestyle choice. It is amusing, and I find myself wondering if I have mistakenly judged other people by their appearance in the past.

The way I see it, I can either wear a hat/scarf/wig, or I can walk confidently with my head held high and let them think what they want. I choose the latter.

Hair Watch—Week Twenty-One

Friday, August 30: When I lost my hair due to chemotherapy, people would tell me that when it grows back, it comes in different from your previous hair (BC—before cancer). What they didn't say was that it could come back different on each side! I used to speculate on what my hair would look like. Curls would be nice. My BC hair was straight and coarse. I thought having hair that was a little thinner or less heavy would be nice. Maybe I would get to try out a new color. Well, I got all of the above.

Gene had a haircut scheduled for Saturday, and I rode along for the fun of it. I walked in and showed Shawn the left, curly side of my hair, and he admired it appropriately and commented on how thick it was coming in. Then I turned to the right (the straight side) and said, "How do you like me now?" He laughed so hard. Then I turned his attention to the top, which is growing straight up. We all laughed. I can laugh because this is Shawn's problem for the next year!

Hair Watch—Week Twenty-Five

Sunday, September 22: I had the best day on Friday. I got the opportunity to work at a fundraiser for a foundation that I sit on the board for. It was a beautiful day, and Tess and I sat at the first hole of a golf course and handed out prizes to golfers. Mostly, we gave the golfers a hard time. Tess and I know nothing about golf, but we were quick to pick up on what the goal is—get as close to the little hole below the flag as possible. With a straight face, we would tell the golfers that they were aiming for the white flag, there was a water hazard on the right, and they should use a driver. All of the golfers took us in stride. It was a fundraiser after all.

The best part of the day was after all the golfers had played through our hole and we were free to explore the course in a golf cart—backward. I'm not sure how that happened or even if it is legal (or encouraged) on golf courses, but Tess was driving, and somehow it made sense at the time. We laughed as she rounded corners on two wheels. The wind was blowing through our hair—well, through Tess's hair—and all was right in the world. It felt incredibly good to be doing something for someone else and not focusing on beating cancer. I have volunteered all of my adult life, and it felt good to get back to it.

A funny opportunity presented itself when we passed one hole and found a photo of my former self promoting the fundraiser. We just could not resist stopping for a photo op. I held up the sign with my smiling former image, and we took what could be a before-and-after photo. The day ended with me giving a speech about the importance of the foundation and all the good that comes from our work. My first speech in over a year. It felt great!

Taking One for the Team

Thursday, September 26: I heard a news story on the radio the other day about Colin Kaepernick shaving off one of his eyebrows after losing his bet with Seahawks quarterback Russell Wilson. Both Russell Wilson and Colin Kaepernick entered the Seahawks-49ers football game having wagered (in a commercial for the new *Madden* video game) their respective eyebrows: the loser of Sunday's big game would have to shave one eyebrow, while the other watched in glory. When the story aired, I turned to Gene and said, "I should send him an e-mail." After all, I lost both eyebrows to chemo, and I know that eyebrows actually have a function and aren't just cosmetic—*and* they take months to grow back. Poor guy. I actually felt sorry for him.

So my husband e-mailed our local radio station to get a link to the story so I could share it—and maybe write Kaepernick a letter. Katheryn Foxx of KKSY (Kiss Country) Radio e-mailed back to say Kaepernick didn't really do it. It was only a publicity stunt. (Sigh.) Now I'm disappointed. Here I was feeling sorry for the guy because I know how hard it is to have people look at you funny. Because of chemo, I have gone without hair for eight months, and I'm just now getting some eyebrows back. Couldn't he at least take one (eyebrow) for the team?

Look at the experiences he is missing out on. When you shower or when it rains, your eyebrows actually direct the water away from your eyes. He could have blamed his red eyes (from crying because he lost the game) on getting soap in his eyes. Without eyebrows, it is nearly impossible to appear surprised. Think of the advantage that would be in press conferences for Kaepernick. "Colin, why did you throw that interception in the second quarter?"

Kaepernick could reply, "That wasn't an interception. I meant to throw it there to make the game more exciting!" Though with only one eyebrow, he might look permanently surprised, in which case he could reply, "I threw an interception?"

It is your loss, Kaepernick. You should have taken one for the team!

Hair Watch—Week Thirty-Two (Perfect!)

Monday, November 18: I go with Gene each month to chat with my hairstylist as he cuts Gene's hair, and we laugh at the progress I have made since my last visit. This month, Shawn declared my hair "perfect" as it is. No stray runaway hairs, no bald spots: just perfect. You have to love positive reinforcement. I would say that my hair is about an inch and a half now, except in the bangs area, which is about a half an inch long. I have some amazing eyelashes though. My eyebrows are about half as thick as they used to be. Don't hold me to this, but I may put a comb on my Christmas list.

It was a year ago that Shawn graciously and kindly shaved my head. I remember my decision to shave my head rather than watch my hair fall out. My doctor had told me that my hair would fall out over Thanksgiving weekend, and I did not want this memory to cloud future holidays. More importantly, I didn't want Gene to have to shave my head for me if all the salons were closed. So I asked Shawn if he would do it before his normal open hours and let my friends come in for support.

Choosing the friends to go with me was important. I needed people I could trust to support me if I laughed or cried or both. I needed people who get my sense of humor and would understand that sometimes it is easier to laugh than cry. Most of all, I needed people who would not treat me like I was fragile or sick. And I needed the best head shaver in the business—because I wanted a Mohawk for a once-in-my-life experience.

It is probably just as well that I did not know how long I would be without hair after that day. It might have been discouraging. But I will always remember the laughter and kindness that was shown to me that day. I would not have chosen to do this any other way.

I have surrounded myself with great friends and family who support me and laugh with me as I make the best of bad hair days. We joke about asking Santa for bangs for Christmas and how much money I have saved on hair products and haircuts. But most of all, they see past the surface and help me celebrate life. Thank you, my friends.

The Einstein Effect

Sunday, February 8, 2014: It has been ten months, and I am starting to see some significant hair growth. In the back, my hair is about three inches long when I stretch the curls out. But the bangs…sigh…the bangs. My bangs continue to grow slowly. If I were to be generous, I would say they are about half the length of too-short bangs. And then there is the "Einstein effect," as I like to call it.

I have never had curly hair, and I admit, I haven't been very sympathetic to people who have complained about curly hair. My theory was that the rest of us spend all our time trying to put curl into our hair, so what do people with curly hair have to complain about? When my hair started coming in curly, I thought, "Yippee for me!" It turns out that curly hair is not maintenance-free.

For several months, I have washed my hair, towel-dried it, and gone on with my life. Boom, I'm done. But as I have started to get some length in my hair, the Einstein effect has taken over. As my hair dries, it starts to grow. It gets bushier and bushier until I look like I have a 1970s afro. By the end of the day, I look like a crazy scientist or Albert Einstein. The only problem is that I don't feel smarter.

As I was talking to a friend about the problem, she told me that I was supposed to use product on it to keep the frizzies away. Who knew? So I went shopping, and I did find some hair paste that tames it in the morning, but by evening, I'm back to the Einstein effect.

I find myself wondering what other people think of my hair. Do they think I went through a catalogue at the beauty salon and said, "I want that one?" Or do they think I have a particularly bad hairstylist? For years, people have asked me who cut my hair, and I have referred them to Shawn. I often tease him that I want to be on commission. But as I think about it, no one has asked me who my stylist is for quite some time. Granted, I was bald for most of a year, but I have hair now. I sort of feel like I should wear a disclaimer that says, "It isn't Shawn's fault!"

The Mirror

Wednesday, April 2: When I first shaved my head, I was always startled when I looked in the mirror. I thought that with time, I would get used to my new reflection and the sight of my bald head, but I never did. I would look into the mirror and not recognize my own reflection. My solution was to avoid looking into the mirror. I was not embarrassed to have cancer or to be bald. I was not embarrassed for people to see me. It was simply unsettling to look at my reflection and not recognize myself.

When my hair started growing back, it was dark and very curly. Not *my* hair. But since I had promised not to complain about hair—considering that any hair was better than no hair—I just washed it and towel-dried it and went on my way. I remember walking up to the microwave one day and seeing a reflection in the glass. It was my grandmother's reflection. She used to go regularly to the hair dresser to get her hair permed and curled tightly. I'm pretty sure they put enough hair spray on it to hold it steady for at least a week. So while it was startling to see my grandmother's reflection (since she passed away many years ago), it made me laugh and think of how she would have laughed when I told her that story.

This week I passed the one-year mark since I stopped taking the chemo. In that year, I would guess that my hair has grown about two to three inches, except for the stubborn bangs area, which is holding out for some sort of incentive. As I mentioned earlier, the additional length has taken on the Einstein effect and sort of grows uncontrollably throughout the day to the point that I look like a mad scientist by the end of the day. I have tried various hair products to try to control it, but it just will not be contained.

So last weekend was my first official, all-over haircut. When Shawn asked me what I was thinking of for a style, I told him that I wanted my hair to look more like a plan and less like a mistake. He laughed. I managed, barely, not to complain about my hair but looked at him pleadingly and said, "Help me!"

Shawn cut, trimmed, walked around me a lot, and then started pulling out his arsenal of products. He applied paste, spray, sticky stuff, and who knows what, then instructed me on the use of a paddle brush. Who knew brushes had names? When he asked if I had a paddle brush, I just looked confused. "Never mind. I'm giving you one," he said. Then he pulled out a flattening iron and asked if I had one of those. Seriously, Shawn. You have cut my hair for twenty years, and you know straightening my hair has not been an issue I have ever faced. I have spent years trying to get it to take a curl. Now I'm trying to tame the curl.

As Shawn finished, he turned my chair to face the mirror, and I didn't know what to say. I looked into the mirror and recognized myself. Sure, the bangs were shorter and the color was different, but the cut and style was similar to my former self. I continued to look at my reflection and said to Shawn, "I don't know what to say. Words can't explain how I feel." How do you thank someone for bringing you back?

Tess visited a few days later, and the first thing she said was, "You look like you again." Woo-hoo!

I Only Got Lost Once

Thursday, Aril 17: Have you ever noticed that whenever you get cocky, it comes back to bite you? Today was one of those days. I traveled with Gene to Minneapolis so he could attend a meeting and I could visit with my old friend: the mall. We arrived a bit early and checked into the hotel. As we left to take Gene to his meeting, he asked me if I knew the name of the hotel and our room number. I promptly responded correctly and smirked at him. No more memory issues for me, boy howdy! Then I correctly drove the three blocks to his meeting location without help. I patted myself on the back as Gene told me to be careful and he would see me in two hours. He actually looked a bit worried.

I shifted the car into D for "Drive me to the mall," and it did. Things were going well, and I managed to make a couple of purchases and find my car again. I couldn't think of anything else I wanted or needed, so I decided to return to the hotel and wait for Gene's meeting to end. I confidently turned onto the street I needed and drove and drove, looking left and right for the hotel sign. I couldn't believe it. Someone had moved the hotel in just one hour! How could that be? As I crossed over I-495 for the second time, I noted that the traffic hadn't improved. Since I didn't plan on getting on the highway, I didn't care. I thought, "Those poor people." They looked tired and aggravated. I, however, was on an adventure.

This was a hard place to navigate, I decided. Sure, the streets were mostly straight and ran straight north and south, or east and west, but there were buildings and cars in the way, and I couldn't seem to get the right combination of turns to find the hotel. The building that Gene was in was constantly on my right, so I knew I was in the right general area. I also knew that I was circling in on my intended location (literally), but it was difficult to land in the right place.

I finally found my hotel and even remembered my room number. Take that, chemo brain. Then I needed to go pick Gene up from his meeting. (I hoped he wouldn't check the odometer.) When he asked how it went, I replied, "I only got lost once!"

Low Memory

Tuesday, June 3: One of my electronic devices flashed a "Low Memory" warning at me last week. Naturally, I thought it was talking about the device, when it turned out it was a forewarning. Just when I think that I'm doing better and chemo brain is fading, I have one of those moments that makes you either laugh or bang your head on the wall.

I called a client Friday morning and reached his voice mail. I left a message and my phone number and hung up the phone. Then I thought, "Hmm. That wasn't my correct phone number. Oops." So I hit redial and left a second message, an apology, and my correct phone number…or so I thought.

Ten minutes later, I got an e-mail from my client saying that neither of the numbers I left seemed to be working. As I looked up the client's phone number (because I couldn't remember it) again, I glanced around my desk for some sort of help in figuring out what my actual phone number was. Surely there must have been some piece of paper in the house that had my phone number on it. I just couldn't seem to figure it out.

The client was very understanding, and we laughed about chemo brain. He said that people who hadn't been through something like this just didn't get it. I knew he would understand as his wife is a breast cancer survivor, so I wasn't worried about looking totally incompetent. We chatted for a while, and then I made him laugh by asking, "Hey, can you tell me what phone number I'm calling from? I want to write it down." My low-memory indicator must have been flashing furiously because all I had to do was pick up my cell phone and look up my home phone number. No wonder Gene worries about me when I drive myself somewhere.

Six-Month Checkup

I had my six-month-postchemo checkup today. It was so exciting. As I arrived at the cancer clinic, I sat in the car and stared at the building for a few minutes thinking about all that I had been through in that building. I thought of all the times I had sat outside and cried, either from sadness, fear, or frustration. And I thought of the tears of laughter as Tess gave some parting shot over the phone to encourage me to charge into the building and take no prisoners. I thought of the many, many infusions, blood tests, radiation treatments, and doctor's appointments I had sat through, and I wondered exactly how many hours I had spent in that building.

I walked into the clinic without my chemo bag and with my real hair in place and wondered if anything had changed in the past six months. I noticed that the hand sanitizers were no longer just inside the doors or at the elevator. I also noted that someone had removed the well-intended but very confusing stickers from the elevator buttons. (Maybe they read my blog!) As I waited to register, I glanced around for the suggestion box that I suggested, but there was no sign of one. Maybe they lost the suggestion.

I gave the registrar a high five when I realized they no longer require a hospital bracelet for patients. I hated wearing the bracelet when I was there. It made me feel like an inpatient. I was always trying to slip it off my wrist just to give the nurses a hard time. Just for fun, we took a new photo for my chart—this one *with* hair. I had my labs drawn and let the lab techs admire my curly hair. We caught up on the past six months, and they said it was so nice to see my smile.

As I waited to see my doctor, I opened the crossword puzzle book that I had worked on during chemo. I was delighted to see that my memory has improved to the point that I could fill in so many more words in the puzzles. I'm not particularly gifted at crossword puzzles, but it was reassuring that many of the missing brain cells have returned in the past six months. Since I could never finish a crossword puzzle before chemo, it would not be fair to expect to finish one now.

My visit with the doctor was easy. We caught up on my reconstruction, travels, and progress on my book. She did a quick physical and looked at my labs and called me "good to go" for another six months. I didn't require any additional tests or procedures. Her parting shot was a reminder that I was overdue for a colonoscopy. Super! I scheduled my one-year checkup for January and left the building with a big smile on my face.

So many people have asked if getting a clean report was a relief, and I have to laugh and say, "No." I was totally confident that this would be an uneventful appointment, but there was a sense of accomplishment that another goal had been reached. I am now a survivor.

Duplicate Gifts

Tuesday, January 13, 2015: Tess and I recently went to visit my mother in Texas. I have been making the trip back and forth to Texas on my own for several years, but both Gene and Tess felt it would be safer if I had a traveling companion. Maybe they were afraid I would end up on the national news as this confused woman wandering the DFW airport, mumbling, "I know I was going somewhere. Now where could that be?" And besides, traveling with Tess is always fun, and she offered to carry my bags, so how could I resist?

While we were at Mom's house, I pulled out some silicone measuring cups and commented that I just loved them. Mom said, "You must, because you gave me two sets." I did? She told me that I had given her a set for the last two Christmases. Not only that, I had given her two sets of personalized coasters as well. Tess chimed in, "I got two sets as well. And two sets of stationery." When I got home and told Danielle the story, she laughed and said, "Mom, you gave everybody the same gifts two years in a row." Well, darn! Why didn't somebody say something?

In my own defense, I don't even remember the last two Christmases. And if you find a great gift, why not give it twice?

CHAPTER 8
RECONSTRUCTION

Friday, September 27, 2013: Many of my friends have asked why I didn't have reconstruction done at the time of my mastectomy. The primary reason is that I was not a candidate for immediate reconstruction, because I was scheduled to have radiation. Radiation can damage or destroy skin tissue, so surgeons want to wait until after radiation to do reconstruction. The second reason is that I wasn't sure if I wanted reconstruction. I needed time to think about my options. Many women choose not to undergo the extra surgery and pain of reconstruction.

So I decided to meet with a plastic surgeon to discuss my options. Gene went through the reconstruction options with me prior to the doctor's visit so that I would be prepared with questions. I found myself very nervous about this appointment because of body image issues. We all have body image issues of some sort, and I know that doctors see patients of all shapes and sizes, but that doesn't make it any easier. When I told Gene that I was nervous, he asked me if I would be more comfortable if he was not in the room during the exam. I said, "Heck no! You are my safety net."

We are escorted to the patient exam room, and I sit in the chair rather than on the exam table. It is my own form of rebellion. I just can't help myself. If there is a chair in the room, I'm taking it rather than the paper-covered table. When you sit on paper, it crackles every time you squirm, and I suspect I will be squirming a lot. The nurse takes my vitals and explains that we will meet the surgeon in his office first, and then he will examine me, measure me, and take photos afterward. Oh boy! More nude photos in my file. I will give the surgeon credit for meeting me with my clothes on first. This consideration always makes an impression on me.

While we wait to meet the doctor, I start looking around the exam room, and I'm disappointed. Gene asks me what I am looking for, and I tell him that I thought there would be more toys to play with. He raises an eyebrow as I explain that in a dermatologist's office, there are photos of moles, poison ivy, sun damage, and so on. I thought there would be charts of noses to choose from, or at least some breast implants lying around, in a plastic surgeon's exam room. He shakes his head. I fidget and sigh.

We are escorted to the plastic surgeon's office. He is very nice and asks Gene where he practices, and they go into a quick back-and-forth while I discreetly look around. Bingo! There are breast implants on the desk. No noses or other props, so I suspect he has prepared specifically for us, and this is not the setup for every patient.

What follows is an oral history of breast augmentation and a number of options available to patients but not necessarily available to me. After about the second or third option and list of potential complications and remedies, I simply can't absorb anymore. The nurse sticks her head in to tell the doctor something, and I lean toward Gene and whisper, "Are you getting all of this?"

He says, "Yes, most of it."

I reply, "Good. I'm lost, and you are in charge of data collection." We have been married thirty years, and delegating responsibility works for us. Ask me about websites or search engine optimization, strategic planning or investments, and I can talk with you for hours. Start discussing medical terms, and I'm pulling out my secret weapon: Gene. It isn't that I won't make the decision for myself; I'm just putting him in charge of collecting and consolidating data.

I'm disappointed to learn that I'm not a candidate for the reconstruction that comes with a free tummy tuck. I should be able to come out of all of this chemo and radiation with some perks. After the discussion, we are moved back to the exam room, where I disrobe. The nurse goes through the process of what would happen during this visit with me one more time, and then the doctor comes in to examine me. He measures things, and I find myself wondering what his reference is for his starting point. The end point of the measuring tape each time seems to be my nipple. But his starting point seems to vary. My sense of humor is raising its ugly head, and I'm not sure the doctor is going to appreciate it. I try to keep my thoughts to myself…mostly.

There is an amusing moment when the surgeon asks my bra size and my mind goes totally blank. Gene tries to be helpful by picking up my bra and finding a size. It turns out that he doesn't know where the size tag is located. The nurse helpfully steps over and finds the size for him. I try not to laugh.

The last indignity is the photo shoot. The surgeon sits on a stool with me standing topless next to a wall. Face forward, snap. Face forty-five degrees, snap. Face sideways, snap. Reverse the process, snap. The best part is that the nurse is standing behind the doctor, and they are pointing in unison to show me which way to face. They look like synchronized flight attendants, and I just have to laugh. It is a nice distraction from the fact that once again, someone is taking photos of my bare chest.

Later in the week, when my oncologist runs into Gene and asks how the appointment went, he replies, "I deserve one-and-a-half hours of CME [continuing medical education], and I think all Kathy heard was white noise." I would say that is a very succinct summary of our visit.

If I do have reconstruction, I'm getting myself a T-shirt that reads: "Hell yes, they are fake. The real ones tried to kill me!"

The Decision

Tuesday, November 12: When I was first diagnosed with breast cancer one year ago, I had to make a lot of decisions about my treatment in a short amount of time. I was understandably frightened, nervous, uncertain, and worried as I worked my way through half a dozen doctor's appointments and listened to their advice. It became clear quite early on that I would not be a candidate for a lumpectomy and would need a mastectomy. But I had to make a decision on whether to remove one breast or two.

My first instinct was to remove both breasts. I had cancer, and it scared me. I wanted it (the cancer) out. Even though the tests said that I didn't have cancer in my left breast, what if they were wrong? But I didn't want to overreact either. After consulting with my surgeon and my husband, I still wrestled with the decision but decided to trust the science and remove only the affected breast. My sweet husband assured me that if I ever changed my mind, I could always have a prophylactic mastectomy done later.

As time wore on, a few things became clear to me:

- First and foremost, I don't ever want to have to go through diagnosis and treatment for breast cancer again. I'm a strong person, but to face this again would be so difficult.
- I don't want to worry for a week before and after my mammogram each year that they will find something. I was surprised at how much that bothered me this year when I went for my annual mammogram. My doctors had assured me that with the amount of chemo they had put into my body, they would be shocked if a radiologist found anything on my X-rays. But I worried anyway.
- The asymmetry of having only one breast is a nuisance. Prosthetics are heavy and hot. And I'm not sure they float, so what if I'm in the pool? Do I wear a prosthetic in my swimsuit or go without?

- I promised my children that breast cancer would not kill me, and I plan to do everything within my power to make this true.
- I'm not feeling particularly lucky.
- And I have exceeded my attention span for being a cancer patient.

With all this in mind, I have decided to have a prophylactic mastectomy done on my left breast later this month. It wasn't an easy decision, but I am at peace with it. I know it is the right thing to do for me. And it turns out that I get choices with this second mastectomy, and I get to have the surgery done at my convenience. I love this!

The first decision I had to make was whether or not to keep the nipple. Let me tell you, this is a fun conversation to have with a stranger (doctor)! My doctor explained that by leaving the nipple, there is a very slight increased risk of cancer, and that there would not be any feeling or sensation to the nipple. So in my mind, what is the point (get it?) of keeping it?

The next decision I had to make was whether or not to have reconstruction done on that side. I met with a plastic surgeon, who described my options, and I decided to have immediate reconstruction following the prophylactic mastectomy. I did ask if he could relocate my breast back to its original position. (I don't think he appreciates my humor yet.) I was advised that I cannot have reconstruction on my right side for another year due to the skin damage from radiation. So we will give the left side a whirl and see how it goes.

The final decision was whether or not I should get nipple tattoos after surgery. I have talked with a number of women about this, as well as my husband. He assured me that it was up to me to decide. So I have made a decision: I'm skipping the tattoos and going straight for stickers instead. Yes, you read correctly. I'm going to get seasonal stickers to use as nipples purely for entertainment. I can change them out each day to match the season or my mood. They won't hurt, and I can laugh as I think about what people don't see. Who says cancer can't be funny!

Surgery Day

Thursday, November 21: Tomorrow is surgery day—finally—and I have run out of things to organize. I get the easy part and get to sleep through the mastectomy and reconstruction and let the doctors do their thing without any input from me. My mom has arrived to help for a week, and Steven flies in to take over "Mommy Day Care" for week two, so I am in good hands. Fingers crossed that I can stay out of trouble at the hospital in the morning and yet still come out with some funny stories. I very much appreciate the calls, notes, and e-mails this week.

Surgery Two

Tuesday, December 3: Surgery is over, and I am home recovering as I reflect on how different this surgery was from my first mastectomy. There was so much fear and uncertainty with the initial diagnosis of cancer and surgery. I could hardly eat or sleep as surgery approached. It was easier this time—and I slept just fine the night before surgery.

I scored the premium time slot for surgery this time: first thing in the morning. Other than having to get up at some awful hour, this is a great time of day to have surgery. Everyone is well rested and ready to go. There are no delays. I am tired, so I don't mind the upcoming nap. And my sense of humor is at its best.

My surgery was scheduled at the competing hospital in town because of the date I chose. It was my first visit to this hospital, so everything was new, and I had lots to entertain me while I waited (for all of five minutes). I pondered the sign that listed the open hours as 4:00 a.m. to 6:00 p.m. I had the first OR time of the day at seven, which meant I had to be there by six. Who has to get there at four in the morning? Ugh!

When I had my preop phone call, I was told the surgery holding area was all private rooms that included their own bathrooms. The nurse on the phone made this seem like a nice selling point. So I had to laugh as we walked into a room you could barely squeeze the four of us into, and the nurse pointed to the toilet in the corner. It was a commode with a fold-down chair on top of it. To use the toilet, you had to fold the chair up and ask everyone to leave the room. Yes, that is special indeed.

My nurse was nice, and we chatted about what to expect in my surgery and recovery. I noticed that everyone was very nice, but no one was treating me like I was fragile like they did when I had my first surgery. I liked that. We discussed the infamous smiley-face pain chart, and she asked me at what level of pain I would ask for pain medicine. I replied eight. She frowned and jotted a note in my chart (and I'm sure I don't want to know what it said). I then explained that no matter what my pain level was, I would always reply three, so the eight that I said earlier was irrelevant. She laughed and asked me why I always said three. I explained that in my mind, they would let me out quicker if I told them my pain level was a three. The nurse told me that I needed to use all my energy on healing and less on fighting pain. My reply: "Nice try." She laughed.

My general surgeon arrived and verified the type of surgery and which side the mastectomy would be on. I told him that if he gave me a Sharpie, I would mark it for him. He promptly reached up and put an X on my left (only) breast. I sighed and told him that I planned to write "Duh" on it. He laughed, but I was truly disappointed. Gene had already nixed my first idea of the morning. I wanted to put a temporary tattoo on the right side to surprise them when they went to prep me in the OR. The only thing that stopped me was his suggestion that it might delay surgery and inconvenience later patients. Boo.

My surgeon then verified that he was removing the nipple. This is generally when my impish sense of humor comes to the surface, and today was no exception. My mom, my husband, and my daughter were in the room, so I paused to consider my reply. Just as he was leaving the room, I said, "I have decided to go with stickers instead." He paused, and I could tell he was debating on how to reply as I grinned at him. He just shook his head and said, "There are lots of choices these days." It's too bad that the patients get to have all the fun with cancer humor and everyone else has to be respectful.

Things went quickly from that point, and I was in recovery in a short (for me) three-and-a-half hours. I remember trying to work out a problem in my head while I was in recovery, but everything was fuzzy. As they moved me to my room, I met up with my family, and then I remembered the problem. "Where's Maggie?" I asked. Shocked and amused faces looked back at me. (Maggie is my mom's dog.) I frowned at them. Are they slow? "She is itchy and needs her medicine," I told them. Gene patted my arm and told me Maggie was at home in Texas. Darn. I like Maggie. My hospital stay would be so much more fun if she came to visit.

Born-On Date

Monday, December 9: One major beer producer has changed their packaging to remove the "best used by" date and replaced it with a "born on" date. I have decided to follow their lead and use a born-on date for my new breasts. Wouldn't it be nice if we could use this on all of our body parts? My new breast's born-on date is November 22. This is the date of my second mastectomy and first step of reconstruction on the left side. I have chosen to have an implant for this side as it is the least complicated method of reconstruction. Plus, it offers ongoing sources of amusement for people with a quirky sense of humor.

I had assumed, prior to meeting with the plastic surgeon, that he would simply remove the breast tissue and put the implant in the remaining pocket of skin. But as it turns out, the implant goes under the muscle so as to give the breast a more natural appearance and feel. In order to stretch the muscle out enough to accept the implant, a tissue expander is placed under the muscle and slowly filled with saline over a three-month period. I find it best not to think about the process too much.

My plastic surgeon was able to immediately add some saline at the time of my surgery. So when I woke up after my surgery, I had a small mound where my breast used to be. That is already better than the other side, so I consider it a positive outcome. I didn't feel any emotional loss or sadness with the loss of the breast. The way I see it, the surgery greatly reduces my risk of cancer on that side, so the mastectomy was a good thing. Plus, I get to relocate my new breast back to where it was located in my twenties. I had two drains that came out of my armpit area and were annoying me. I hate drains. Ask any patient that has had them, and they will all complain about them. Fortunately, the first one was removed four days after surgery. The second one was removed about ten days after surgery.

I was provided a compression bra to wear day and night for four weeks. Let me tell you, "compression bra" is simply a nice phrase for "corset." This bra has hooks and a zipper in front and Velcro on the shoulders and cinches you in tightly. I find myself pulling on it constantly. They provided me with two of these garments, so I don't even have an excuse to not wear it.

I left the hospital with dire warnings not to lift my arm beyond sixty degrees for the next four weeks. Here are some of my other restrictions:

- Do not lift anything more than ten pounds.
- Rest often.
- No strenuous exercise.

And my favorite,

- Do not do hard work.

I had the nurse highlight that one!

The Filling Station

Friday, December 13: Two weeks after my surgery, it was time for my first fill-up. The tissue expander that was placed under my muscle resembles an empty balloon. Over the next few months, the doctor will slowly fill the expander until it reaches the desired size. There is a port for access, and the doctor has a cool locator tool that finds the port. He calls it a stud finder, and that makes me laugh.

I admit that I was a bit nervous about my first fill-up. I have been on the Internet (I build websites for a living, so of course I was on the Internet!) and read that many patients find the fill-ups painful or uncomfortable. But I was also looking for new material for my blog, and this seemed like a wonderful opportunity for inspiration.

The doctor walked into the room carrying four large syringes. When I say large, I'm talking turkey baster size. The nurse followed with another bottle of saline. I took one look and said, "You are being rather overly optimistic, don't you think?" The doctor quickly hid two of the syringes behind his back and tried to look innocent as his nurse followed suit. Gene and I started laughing. Gene murmurs, "Good one. Throw him off balance as soon as he walks into the room!" I recognize sarcasm when I hear it. (Tess says that Gene says a prayer every day thanking God that I'm not *his* patient.)

The doctor commented that it was natural to be scared at the first fill-up, but that most patients don't find them that bad. I lay back on the table, and he removed the Steri-Strips over my incision. I didn't feel a thing. Then he used his handy locator tool to find my port and asked if I was ready. He inserted the needle into my port, and I didn't feel anything at all. So far so good! Chemo infusions were worse than this. Before I had time to process what was happening, he was already emptying one syringe into my tissue expander. I barely felt my skin move. Then he injected the second syringe, and I felt my chest tighten, but it wasn't painful. About the time I considered saying, "Uncle," he was done.

When I sat up, I definitely felt a fullness in my chest. I was a little achy and my chest felt tight, but I would not call it painful. I was amazed to see that I had grown nearly a full cup size in less than a minute. How cool is that? The doctor stood back and looked at my chest. He seemed happy with the results.

Then we discussed the radiation damage on the other side, and I decided to ask the question that had been worrying me. I asked him if there was a chance that he could not reconstruct my right side. He told me that there were new methods of dealing with severely damaged skin and that he would probably schedule me for hyperbaric treatments sometime next year. He estimated that I would have twenty treatments in the hyperbaric chamber. I glanced at Gene and tried not to laugh.

Gene and I barely made it to the elevator before we doubled over laughing. The thought of putting me in a hyperbaric chamber even once had us in stitches. I'm a bit claustrophobic, and I get bored easily. A confined space for a long period of time is not a good combination for me. But think of all the blog material I could gather!

When we got in the car, Gene gave me a choice. He would either get me some ibuprofen and pick up dinner, or he would take me to an early dinner and I could have a martini. I took one for the team and went for the martini. I felt no pain or discomfort as I sat and sipped my drink. Which got me to thinking: maybe I could have a martini before going into the hyperbaric chamber!

Chicken Wings

Friday, December 20: I had my one-month-postop follow-up appointment with my doctor today, and he lifted my restrictions. I feel like a free woman. For the past month, I have had limited movement of my arm. I could not move it more than sixty degrees or lift anything heavier than ten pounds. This doesn't seem like a big deal, but it results in shoulder and back aches, as well as limiting my ability to reach out and close the car door. I think I may have been restricted from driving as well, but that didn't work out for me, so I ignored it.

As I was walking out and talking to the nurse, she cautioned me to start moving my arm gradually and not go overboard. Do you think nurses have special talents in identifying which patients they need to say this to? I tried to look innocent and nod my head, but I knew exactly what I was going to do when I hit the parking lot: I was going to do the chicken dance! How could I resist?

Just picture me out in the parking lot with the weather at two degrees doing the chicken dance. Woo-hoo for me! For the past month, I have worried about slipping on the ice and putting my arm out to catch myself, only to tear my incision and muscle. I don't believe in do-overs, so I have been unusually cautious this past month, and it is time to spread my wings. Oh, the joy of it. All I needed was some music. As the cold weather started seeping in, I paused to wonder if implants can freeze. Wouldn't it be a hoot trying to explain that one to my doctor?

When Gene got home, I said, "Look what I can do!" and I flapped my wings. His reply was, "Congratulations." I was expecting a more enthusiastic reply, but he did laugh as I caught his eye all evening and raised my eyebrows and flapped my wings. I have certainly learned to celebrate the small things.

The Doctor's Note

Thursday, January 30, 2014: When I was first diagnosed with breast cancer, the doctors said, "You are young, and we want to treat this aggressively." I would respond, "Could I have a doctor's note that says I'm young?" Generally, the doctor would smile or laugh and then move on to important medical information. But I was serious. In my mind, I could see a framed piece of artwork that held doctor's notes that said I was young and that could also get me out of work. I'm not beyond taking advantage of an illness.

I once had a minor day surgery, and as I was packing up to leave, the nurse went over instructions and restrictions. "Don't drive or operate any heavy machinery or make legally binding decisions for the next twenty-four hours. Your judgment will be impaired," she said. Well, my friends will tell you that my judgment was already impaired when I walked into the hospital, even more so after anesthesia. So I asked the nurse if I could have a note saying that I was not allowed to cook for two days. She laughed and promptly wrote the note on my discharge instructions. I could not wait for

Gene to pick me up at the door and show him my note.

I now have made a habit of trying to get doctor's notes whenever possible. It turns out that this note is totally worthless unless you are in high school and trying to get out of PE, but it is fun to see what I can get away with. About midway through radiation, I met with my radiologist, and she examined my skin and told me that I would need to start to limit my activities. A light bulb went off in my mind. When opportunity knocks, I'm ready to open the door! "Does that mean I can't mow?" I asked her with a straight face. She hesitated, then asked how big our yard was. I told her that we had fourteen acres.

Her eyes got big, and she said, "There is no way you can mow that much."

I said, "I'm going to need a note." I love it. I now have a note that says I can't mow. Not that Gene would expect me to anyway, but it is fun to have it in writing.

I pretty much got out of mowing for the summer, so it was time to work on a note for snowplowing and getting out of cooking Thanksgiving dinner. I scheduled my second mastectomy to fall the Friday before Thanksgiving and flew my mother and son Steven up to help me (and, by the way, cook Thanksgiving dinner). The nurses at the hospital covered me with a note that got me out of cooking for at least a week, but I still needed to work on the snow removal issue. So when I went in for my follow-up with the plastic surgeon, I asked if I could have a note that said I couldn't snowplow…for the entire winter. My surgeon wasn't buying it. No note, but he did caution me not to use my arm for four weeks.

I'm out of doctor's notes, and the snow just keeps falling. Maybe I should have asked for a note that says I'm required to go south for healing.

I'm Full

Friday, February 7: After several trips to the plastic surgeon's office, I can now say that I'm full (or full of it). My tissue expander has been injected with saline to the point that I'm satisfied with the result. It turns out that deciding on when you are "full" isn't as scientific as I expected it to be. When I was told that I would have a tissue expander, I thought that the doctor would ask me what bra cup size I wanted to be and he would pull out a chart and say, "You need this number of ccs of saline injected over the next three visits." Not so much.

Each week or two, I have gone into the surgeon's office, and he has injected a couple of tubes of saline into a port in my tissue expander. After injecting the saline into the expander, the surgeon would have me stand before a full-length mirror, and we would all examine the result. Then I would turn to the side, and we would all take another good look and discuss whether we were happy with the result yet, or if I needed more fill. At first I felt self-conscious with a doctor and nurse standing behind me as we looked at my topless reflection in the mirror. Then, bizarrely, it became normal. Does this mean I'm going to become an exhibitionist in the future?

I found that I am a terrible judge when it comes to deciding when enough is enough. Sometimes the doctor would help by saying, "I think you need more." That made it easier. After all, he is a professional, he should be able to help me with this. Other times, I would come home and ask Gene what he thought. Gene was always so considerate and would respond, "That is entirely up to you." While I appreciate the consideration, I don't think any of these people realized that I was truly looking for guidance. When I am done with reconstruction, I don't want to look out of proportion. But I don't want to be large busted either.

Before my last appointment, I decided that I needed a girl's opinion. After failed attempts to meet up with my daughter or friends before my final fill-up, I decided to ask the nurse. She has been nice to me in the past. We had an amusing moment when we pulled my shirt tightly across my bustline and then decided I needed just a bit more fill.

As the nurse set up the equipment, she asked me what it felt like to get a fill. She said that patients often asked her about it and she hadn't experienced it personally. I thought this was a great question since I had read all sorts of horror stories on the Internet before I had surgery. I told her that I hadn't felt the needle in the first visit, but as the feeling was coming back to my chest area over time, I felt the needle prick a bit more each time. It isn't a bad pain, just noticeable.

When the doctor injects the first syringe of saline into my expander, I don't feel anything. As he injects the second syringe, I start to feel some movement under the skin and a tightness. The doctor watches closely to make sure we aren't stretching the skin too quickly or too much. When I sit up after the injections, I feel a significant heaviness and tightness in the breast area. It isn't painful and sort of reminds me of the tenderness in your breasts with PMS. For me, the breast area feels tight for about twenty-four hours. Then it goes away. I have read that other people find these fills more uncomfortable than that, but for me, it isn't painful. It could be because I'm so amused to watch my chest grow as the saline is injected.

After we finished my last fill, my surgeon explained that we could set up my surgery to remove the tissue expander and put in my permanent implant. He also said that we could begin reconstruction on the right side in a few months. I have elected to do both surgeries at the same time to avoid having two surgeries within a couple of months. In the meantime, I am meeting with the wound-healing department to discuss hyperbaric-chamber treatments to treat the radiation damage to the skin on my right chest. Oh boy!

CHAPTER 9
HYPERBARIC OXYGEN THERAPY

The Hyperbaric Chamber

Friday, February 14, 2014: I stand behind my belief that doctors spend their spare time dreaming up additional tests and procedures they can put you through. My plastic surgeon has decided that I need hyperbaric-chamber treatments to treat the skin on my chest and prepare it for reconstructive surgery. My radiation treatments damaged the skin on my chest to where it is thin and no longer very flexible. I'm told that hyperbaric treatments have proven to help heal wounds and damaged skin.

I tried to keep an open mind when the time came to meet with the hyperbaric specialist. But let's face it: I'm claustrophobic and I know it. I can't imagine a good outcome to this appointment. A nurse came in and took my vital signs and promised a tour if I behaved myself. Then the doctor came into the room and discussed the benefits of hyperbaric treatments. He told me that they like to do twenty treatments before surgery and ten to twenty treatments after surgery if my insurance approves the treatment. Since my insurance sucks, I'm thinking I won't get approved for the full thirty treatments, so I give myself a quick high five and thank the insurance gods.

Each hyperbaric treatment is called a "dive" and lasts two to two-and-a-half hours. The doctor tells me that they are given once a day, five days a week. I gulp. The doctor then explains that sometimes the skin heals a bit faster than they anticipate, so I shouldn't worry about those last couple of treatments. Is he kidding? I'm worried about the first couple of treatments, not the last ones!

I tell the doctor that I'm a bit claustrophobic and don't do well in tight spaces. He tells me that most patients don't have a problem in the chamber but they can give me something to lessen my anxiety if I like. The longer he talks to me, the bigger my eyes are getting. When the nurse mentions that it takes twenty-two minutes to get me out of the chamber in case of an emergency, I have visions of myself freaking out and looking for ways to undo some bolts to let myself out. What are the chances I can sneak a screwdriver or one of those emergency glass-break tools in with me?

The doctor then explains that hyperbaric treatments are generally very safe. The main concern is fire. What? The nurse helpfully chimes in that most of the fires are not in this country. Well, I'm reassured. How about you? The doctor agrees with the nurse and says that most fires are in other countries and the only ones in the United States were due to equipment malfunctions. I hear this voice in my head: "It takes twenty-two minutes to get you out of the chamber in case of an emergency." I'm thinking it is a good thing they took my blood pressure at the start of the visit and not right now.

I'm not going to let the doctor have all the fun, so I tell him that I have had some issues with perforated eardrums on commercial flights and that I'm concerned about my ears in the chamber. Why should I be the only one who is worried, right? I have consulted with my ear, nose, and throat doctor, who offered to put tubes in my ears if there was a problem. The specialist decides we should go ahead and put the tubes in my ears before I start treatment. Oh goodie, another procedure.

I must be looking chalky by now because the doctor tells me that he is going to prescribe Valium for me to take before the first treatment. Uh-oh. I clear my throat and say, "I have a little problem with Valium. I tend to interrogate people when I take it."

The doctor starts laughing and says, "That's okay." No, it isn't! I have taken Valium exactly twice in my life, both times for medical procedures, and might I point out, both times were with the same doctor, who should have known better after the first time.

The first time I had Valium, I interrogated my poor doctor about where he went to school, why he chose his specialty, every place he had lived, why he changed specialties, and I probably asked him his grade point average. When I had to have a second procedure done, I tried to talk the doctor out of giving me Valium. I told him I wasn't nervous and probably didn't need it, but oh no, he just had to insist that I take the Valium. "We find that patients do better when they take Valium," he said. Gene went with me to the second procedure, and the doctor let him come into the procedure room since he is also a physician.

Let me tell you, if it came into my head, it came out of my mouth. I asked one question after another and rarely waited for a reply. At one point, I looked over, and Gene was staring at me like he didn't know who I was.

"Why are you looking at me like that?" I asked. "Don't you look at me that way." The really awful part is that I remember the entire thing. So I'm thinking that taking Valium and being confined to a clear tube for two-and-a-half hours is not going to go well.

The doctor leaves the room, and it is time for my tour. As the nurse and I walk toward the chambers, she tells me there is no way she could ever do these treatments. Me either, sister! When we reach the room where the chambers are located, she asks me to wait outside while she goes in to ask the patients if it is okay for me to view the chambers. When we walk into the room, I swear it is like the movie *Coma*. You remember the scene where all the coma patients are suspended from the ceiling in long rows? Except here, there are only two patients in long, clear tubes. One elderly lady turns on her side and waves at me. I think I may have whimpered as I waved back.

I have read that there are two different types of hyperbaric chambers. One is designed for small groups of people and is more like a small room, but most hospitals have gone to the single system that holds one patient at a time. I call them "one-holers." The one-holer is about seven feet long but not tall enough for you to sit up in during treatment. My hospital has two of these chambers, so they can let two patients dive at the same time. A television screen is mounted above each chamber so you can amuse yourself while you dive.

The nurse explains that the lights in the room are turned off to help prevent seizures in the patients. There is that voice in my head again telling me that it takes twenty-two minutes to get me out. I am told that at one point in my dive, I will be asked to wear an oxygen mask. My claustrophobia meter is in the red zone. But I'm told that I will never be alone. A nurse sits with the patients and can hear everything they say. I imagine her turning down the volume as I scream and beg to be released. This makes me snicker.

The nurse tells me that I will have to remove all clothing, jewelry, and so on and wear a hospital gown while in the chamber, and that I cannot take anything, not even a piece of paper, in with me due to risk of fire. I am told not to wear any cosmetics, cologne, shampoo, deodorant, or anything else like that because of that same fire issue. (There goes that voice in my head again!) The chambers are starting to look a lot like coffins. Fortunately, no friends or family are allowed in the dive area, so there won't be any witnesses if I freak out.

The last thing the nurse asks me as I'm preparing for my escape is if I am planning any travel during the treatment time. I tell her that I currently didn't have any travel plans. "Good," she says, "because you can't fly and dive in the same day." I cock my head. Now there is a phrase that I haven't used before and probably won't get to use again in my lifetime. I'm really hoping that someone asks me to take a trip in April so I can reply, "I'm sorry I can't go. I can't fly and dive in the same day."

Truth Serum

Friday, March 7: I had a minor procedure done this week at the community hospital where my husband works. I needed ear tubes to be inserted so that I could start my hyperbaric-chamber treatments. I have a lot of scar tissue in my ears from frequent ear infections, and the doctors were worried that my eardrums would not be able to tolerate the dives properly, so we placed ear tubes as a precaution. This is a procedure that can be done in the office, but I have had it done in the past and it hurt significantly, so I elected to have it done in the operating room.

I took comfort in the fact that I was scheduled to receive general anesthesia. My theory is that if I was totally knocked out, I would be less "helpful" in the OR. On the day of surgery, my surgeon (not my husband in this case, but a close friend) decided all I needed was IV sedation. In my own defense, at this point I started asking every nurse that I came into contact with to please put a pillow over my head if I started talking in the OR. They patted my arm and laughed and reassured me they would be there for me, but I don't think they meant it. I was serious.

The nurse injected half the dose of Versed before we left for the OR. I told her I could already feel it, and she laughed. I do remember her telling me at one point to stop being so helpful and let them take care of me. I know I was messing with the IV, but it was so interesting that I just couldn't resist. I was wheeled to the OR, and the surgeon walked in, and I received the second half of my sedation. This is where my nurse friends failed me. They had a pillow and they didn't use it.

I will say that I felt very clearheaded at the time and *very* comfortable—a bad combination, as it turns out. I greeted my surgeon with, "Hi, Fritz [his nickname]. Do you mind if I call you Fritz in the OR? I would never disrespect you in the OR, and I really do respect you, you know." He paused and smiled at me, and a little voice in my head said, "Time to shut up"—but I didn't.

I don't remember everything clearly, but apparently I had an issue on my mind and requested a meeting with the head of anesthesia. In the preop instructions, I was asked to remove all fingernail and toenail polish before surgery. I took issue with this. Normally, I take issue only at home, but on this day, I decided to go global. As I removed my perfectly good manicure the morning of surgery, I complained to Gene about this unnecessary step. His response? "Take it up with the head of anesthesia. They set the preop rules." I suspect he was just blowing me off, but in my hazy Versed-induced state, it sounded like good advice.

Unfortunately, on this day, my friend Brad, the head of anesthesia, was not working, and New Guy was filling in. New Guy was a good sport as I quizzed him on whether he was the head of anesthesia on this particular day. He promised to schedule a meeting for me with the "real head of anesthesia" at a later date. Since I was making progress, I decided to ask for a doctor's note that said I couldn't snowplow for twenty-four hours. New Guy quickly offered to write me a note *and* to write a note to the head of surgery (my husband) that I should be able to get a new manicure and pedicure, PRN (as needed). This sounded like an excellent idea, and I remember feeling very satisfied.

I'm not sure when my surgeon managed to get any work done without my help, but I do remember one of the nurses commenting that they had never had such a happy patient who smiled all through surgery. Why wouldn't I be smiling? I had enough Versed in me that I'm surprised I didn't ask the surgeon to train me on how to put in ear tubes so I could do it myself next time. All I know is that I knew everyone in the room, and I was feeling a little too comfortable to have my normal brain-to-mouth filters going.

I would like to think this was all a bad dream, but I have the documentation to prove it. I was so proud of my two doctor's notes and couldn't wait to show them to Gene when he got home. He laughed so hard. I don't know how long it will be before I can show my face at the hospital.

My doctor's notes read:

- Is able to return to work when she pleases. No snow removal until she feels ready.
- Can obtain manicure & pedicure, billed to head of surgery at Virginia Gay Hospital, as often as she likes.

My First Dive

Tuesday, March 18: Yesterday was my first hyperbaric-chamber treatment, and I will admit that I was anxious about how I would do. I tried to follow my mother's advice and not think about it too much, but the combination of a confined space and Valium had me worried. Fortunately, I was scheduled for late afternoon, so Gene was able to arrange his schedule so he could go with me.

As soon as we pulled out of the driveway, I opened the container of Valium and took one pill. The label said to take one to two pills thirty minutes prior to arriving at the hospital. Having prior experience with Valium, I decided to take just one pill. I then turned to Gene and said, "I'm sorry." He told me not to worry about it because lots of patients have to take Valium before procedures. I laughed and said, "I'm not apologizing for taking the Valium. I'm apologizing for anything I might say or do once it takes effect!" He laughed with me.

As we neared the hospital, I could feel the effects of the Valium. I decided that God has a great sense of humor because as we took the downtown exit, we saw tons of green people walking around in odd costumes. It turns out that it was Saint Patrick's Day, and the Saint Paddy's Day parade was just letting out. Gene dodged all types of green characters as I tried to focus. I stumbled over words and phrases as I tried to tell Gene a story. He was very helpful when we got into the hospital elevator, and I leaned in to stare at the elevator panel and tried to make up my mind on which button to push. My mind was fuzzy, and I felt like I was grinning a lot.

As I checked in, there were two nurses, and each asked me a question. I told them they were going to have to slow down because I was premedicated and having difficulty following the conversation. Then I grinned at them and asked, "Did you ask me a question?" There was a brief discussion about my port, and I was just proud that I remembered that I had one. But they were asking me for details, and I couldn't focus, so I just shrugged my shoulders. I seemed to have missed the significance of their questions.

As we sat in the waiting room, my doctor and nurse came out and once again started questioning me about my port. It seems that safety protocol says that they have to call the manufacturer to make sure my port is safe in the hyperbaric chamber. The doctor asked if I had been given a card with the name of the company that manufactured my port and the model and serial number of my particular port. I assured him that I had indeed been given a card like that. "Do you have it with you?" he asked.

"Nope," I replied. I told them I was sure it would be fine and we should just go ahead and get started. Gene just shook his head. The doctor asked if I had taken my Valium. "Yes, and I brought the whole bottle just in case." The warning on the prescription bottle reads: "Taking this medication alone or with alcohol may lessen your ability to drive or perform hazardous tasks." I think they should add "or make safety decisions." Fortunately, I was not in charge of safety protocol.

Gene was helpful and started going through my wallet to look for the card since I seemed to be having trouble focusing. At some point he reminded me that I had cleaned out my wallet prior to our vacation and put all the nonessentials in a safe place, and apparently my port card didn't make the cut. I told Gene that I knew *exactly* where the port card was (a big fat lie). Since I was of no help, one of the nurses called the operating room department, and they were able to pull my chart and find the manufacturer and serial number and call the company and get assurance that my port would be safe.

Meanwhile, Gene asked me what I was thinking about so hard. I told him that I was trying to figure out a way of escaping. He laughed. In fact, I had just remembered that I meant to bring a note to give to the nurses to tell them "I'm not normally this way." I was trying to figure out where I could get some paper and a pen.

I was finally cleared to dive, taken to the dressing room, and instructed to remove all my clothing and my eyeglasses and change into the designer hospital gown. No socks, no underwear, nothing but my birthday suit. No books, no phones, no smoking materials (duh!), nothing flammable. There were big charts on the walls listing the things you could not take with you on your dive, but without my glasses, they were just fuzzy photos.

The nurse took my vitals and went through a checklist to make sure I wasn't trying to sneak anything in with me. With the caution that they didn't want anything to spontaneously combust while I was in the chamber, I wasn't taking any chances. I was covered with two hospital blankets and handed a water bottle (maybe this was so I could put out any fires?) and an oxygen mask. Neither of these items comforted me. In fact, when the nurse cautioned me to keep the lid open on the water bottle so it wouldn't explode during my dive, the wheels in my brain started turning. That sounded like fun. Then she had me practice using my oxygen mask. Claustrophobia raised its ugly head, and I wasn't even in the chamber yet. The nurse told me if I got nauseated or light headed, to just use the oxygen mask and I would be breathing normal room air and it would help. The logic escaped me, but I nodded my head.

The nurse asked if I was ready, then pushed me halfway into the chamber. The Valium was doing its job, and I hadn't started crying or pleading for my release yet. At this point, she put an elastic band on my arm and explained that it was a grounding wire. What? That didn't sound good. I was then instructed to push a button to verify that I was indeed grounded. That didn't sound like a good idea either, especially when I failed the test. After jiggling the wristband a few times, I was finally able to pass the grounding test. I was not reassured. I'm thinking I should have paid more attention in science class when they explained how electricity works.

The nurse pushed me the rest of the way into the chamber and softly closed the door. I tried not to imagine a bank vault closing with me on the inside. She immediately picked up the phone and started talking to me in a reassuring voice. I had a death grip on my oxygen mask and water bottle and stared worriedly at my grounding wire. She said, "Here we go." We? How about *we* trade places, and you let me know how we are doing?

I heard a fan start up, and the chamber immediately began to smell like warm, humid chlorinated water. I told the nurse that it smelled like an indoor pool. She explained that they sanitize the inside of the chamber with chlorine bleach between patients. I wondered if bleach was flammable. I decided to pretend I was at the pool instead of being stuck in a one-holer. My right ear began to pop immediately, and I was glad that we went ahead and put ear tubes in.

The inside of the chamber is a bit roomier than it looks from the outside. There is room to move your arms around and wiggle your feet. With some effort, you can actually bend your knees and rest your feet on the mattress to give your back some relief. I'm a fidgeter, so I wiggled and shifted often and tried to not think about escaping.

Since I was allowed to bring DVDs with me, I took the first season of *Downton Abbey* with me to keep me entertained. Because the chamber is a cylinder, looking through it to watch television is similar to looking through a prism. The images on the TV were a bit blurred and distorted, so I entertained myself by shifting now and then to watch the people sway like the reflection in one of those carnival mirrors. When the first episode ended, I prayed that it was a two-hour episode rather than one hour, because I could not imagine spending another hour in the chamber. Unfortunately, my prayers were not fruitful. I did get a kick out of looking through the chamber and seeing the nurses and doctor watching the TV with me for a few minutes.

When I was finally released from the chamber, it was half past five, and I could not wait to get out of the hospital. There was no happy buzz left from the Valium, and I had had enough confinement for the day. Gene looked like he had been through the ringer as much as I had. He told me that some patient had tuned the waiting room television to a marathon of *Criminal Minds*.

Gene told me that he was very impressed with their safety concerns and making sure my port was not going to be an issue. Then he mentioned that he was surprised they weren't more concerned about my temporary implant since it was filled with saline. I told Gene about the nurse's warning about my water bottle and asked him if he could imagine my implant growing larger under pressure and then exploding, and we both started laughing. I will have to ask the doctor about it on my next dive. I can't believe I'm actually going to go back.

Pride Goeth before the Fall

Tuesday, March 25: I have received a number of e-mails from people asking exactly what would happen if I did freak out in the hyperbaric chamber. I have to admit this question makes me laugh at the possibilities. I have given considerable thought to exactly what would happen if I freaked out while in the tube. After all, I'm stuck in the clear cylinder for over two hours each weekday, and I have to occupy my mind with something.

I'm really not the type to start screaming, pulling my hair out, and pounding on the Plexiglas walls, though sometimes I wish I were like that. It would be cathartic to just let loose and have a hissy fit now and then. But me? No, I have too much pride and always worry about making a scene. I think the only way that would happen is if they put me in the hyperbaric chamber…with a snake. Then all bets would be off, and there would be one big mess to clean up. (I told you I have a lot of time to think in that tube!)

I feel that if the worst happened and I simply could not stand to be confined in the chamber any longer, I would probably just start crying and beg to be released. And if it truly takes twenty-two minutes to get me out of there, that is a lot of crying. I would probably have one heck of a headache.

Since I survived my first dive in my Valium-induced happy state, I decided to be a big girl and try to do my second dive without any medication assistance. My theory was that the chamber was a bit roomier than I originally feared, and I survived my first dive without freaking out, so how bad could it be? So on dive number two, I drove myself to the hospital and didn't take any Valium. I will admit, I felt pretty anxious about the dive knowing it would be even longer than the previous day.

I can tell you right now that I knew I had made a mistake the instant they closed the door on the chamber. Once again, I clutched my oxygen mask in one hand and my water bottle in the other hand. I looked pleadingly at the nurse as she turned the dial and set my timer. "Please don't do this to me," I was thinking. But I have a lot of pride, and I just couldn't bring myself to knock on the Plexiglas and beg for release. I focused on my breathing and tried to control my heart rate. I vaguely remembered a warning to "never hold your breath," so I started breathing too fast. I could hear Gene's voice in my head: "Slow, steady breaths. You are going to be okay." I pictured myself freaking out in all sorts of ways and what the nurses would say to Gene when they called and asked him to pick me up from the psych ward. But I truly didn't want to cause a scene, so I stuck it out for two-and-a-half hours. When they opened the door, you have never seen anyone get off of a gurney so fast. I didn't care that my gown was backless.

When the doctor came in and asked how it went, I said, "Fine." Big fat liar. But I do have some pride and didn't want to admit to weakness and fear. That evening, Gene asked me how it went, and I was honest with him. "I would rather shoot off my big toe than go back." Here was a great chance for him to laugh, but instead he sympathized with me and asked if I should consider taking the prescribed Valium before the next dive. Since I'm always a negotiator, I asked what he thought about me taking half of a Valium (a quarter of the prescribed dose). I explained that when I take two pills (the prescribed dose), I interrogate people. When I tried taking one pill, I sat with a big grin on my face and had no regard for safety features. So I was thinking half a pill ought to be just right. We agreed that it was a good plan.

So on dive number three, I swallowed half a pill when I got to the hospital parking lot. It turns out that for me, half a pill is the magic dose. I'm still somewhat sane and rational, but I can go into the chamber without grasping the rim and pleading for a pardon.

Amphitrite—Queen of the Sea

Saturday, April 5: I have now completed thirteen hyperbaric (HBO) chamber dives and now consider myself Amphitrite—Goddess Queen of the Sea! I found this description of Amphitrite on the Theoi Greek Mythology website, and it made me laugh: "Amphitrite was the goddess queen of the sea, but most simply describe her as the female personification of the sea: the loud-moaning mother of fish, seals, and dolphins." That is exactly how I feel—loud moaning. My friends are asking me if it is getting any easier. My response: "Hell no! I'm pretty sure that I'm losing my mind." I can tell you that I have completed the entire series of *Downton Abbey*. If you have any questions, just let me know.

It should come as no surprise that since the novelty of getting to watch unlimited movies and television has worn off, I have found other ways to amuse myself during treatment. Since I'm allowed to take only a fire extinguisher (my water bottle) and an oxygen mask into the chamber with me, my options for entertainment are limited. I have inspected, disassembled, and reassembled my oxygen mask, and it no longer holds much entertainment value. Sometimes I try to suction it to my forehead or cheek, and once, when the nurse wasn't looking, I tried to stick it to the roof of the chamber and see if it would hold. When I get really bored, I start talking into it like I'm a pilot.

The water bottle got me into trouble last week. My movie had ended, so I started inspecting my water bottle and squeezing it to watch the water rise, then letting go to watch the water level fall. I squeezed a bit too hard, and water shot out the top and sprayed the top of the HBO chamber. The nurse was startled and looked up. My eyes were huge, and then I started laughing. She picked up the phone and asked what had happened. I so wish I had thought to say that my implant had exploded! But I just shrugged and laughed and started mopping the top of the chamber with my blanket. She told me she was going to send in a cleaning rag on my next dive.

I have found a way to bend my knees and do small leg lifts in the chamber. With some work, I can get my arm behind my head. A friend of mine went through HBO when he had his leg amputated, and he told me that with enough time, he got to where he could roll over on his stomach. My imagination ran wild as I considered exactly how a person would accomplish this. Then I considered a fish flopping around on the bank of a river, and I think this must be how he managed to roll over. It gives me a goal to work toward.

One of my nurses told me that most people try to take a nap while in the chamber. I told her that I could never sleep in there. She asked me why. I explained that if I woke up in there, I would think I was in a coffin and would start searching frantically for that string that is hooked to a bell. She wasn't familiar with "safety coffin" bells but started laughing as I explained the concept to her. "Safety coffins included some type of device for communication to the outside world, such as a cord attached to a bell that the person could ring should he revive after the burial." So I keep my eyes open while in the chamber...just in case. And the nurses wonder why my heart rate is so high when I go into the chamber!

Seven more dives to go before surgery and ten dives after surgery. That is something like seven dog years. I have been on more dives than most people get to experience in their lives, and I'm hoping to be dive certified when I'm done.

MacGyver (without the Paper Clip)

Tuesday, April 8: As I was spending my two hours in the HBO chamber today, I wondered what MacGyver would do in my situation. If you remember the *MacGyver* television series, whenever MacGyver was stuck in a situation, he would take a paperclip, a lost penny, and the Band-Aid off his thumb and build a lunar module to drive him to the nearest town. I am certain that he would never have spent two hours in the HBO chamber waiting for someone to open the door for him.

I looked around the chamber and at my two designated toys—the water bottle and oxygen mask—and plotted my escape. What would MacGyver do? The oxygen mask has a small cushion that has been filled with water so it won't explode under pressure. This might work as a life preserver for a hamster in a real-life dive, but it would probably just be messy if I tried to remove it. The hose that connects the mask to the room-oxygen outlet on the door shows some real potential, but it is barely long enough to wrap around my neck, and I'm saving that for when I really can't stand it anymore. There appears to be some sort of paper or fibrous filter in the oxygen mask, and I pause briefly to wonder if it is flammable and, if so, how it got by the safety police who practically frisk me and check crevices before I go in for a dive. And as I have mentioned in the past, I'm saving the water bottle as my emergency fire extinguisher, so I'm not sacrificing it.

I am left with two blankets, a sheet, and a hard pillow. I could unravel the blankets and tear the sheets into strips and form some sort of rope, but I just can't come up with how that would be helpful. The pillow has intrigued me from the start. I just can't figure out what it is made of that wouldn't be flammable so that it is safe to go in with me. It isn't feathers, and it isn't air, but I don't know what is inside. Just for kicks today, I wiggled and fidgeted and slid to the side and was able to get the pillow out from behind my head and onto my stomach. When the nurse looked up, I pretended to be engrossed in the movie. With my eyes glued to the television, I gently poked and prodded the pillow to see if I could find any use for it.

Unfortunately, I still don't know what it is made of, and I had to spend the rest of my dive with no pillow under my head. I ended up sliding it down to my feet and just pretended that was my plan from the start. Oh, if I only had a paperclip!

The Contraband Interrogation

Tuesday, April 15: Prior to each HBO treatment, I am asked if I have any banned items on me or if I have used any products that could be flammable. Posters are placed around the room with images of contraband. The nurse reads a list of questions to which I am supposed to respond no. While they tell you this is a safety check, now that I have seventeen dives out of the way, I'm starting to form my own opinions about why they don't want you to take these items into the chamber with you. I think they are just mean-spirited and don't want you to have any fun while you are lying in one position for two hours, and they certainly don't want you to have any tools to assist in your escape.

The contraband list questions include:

- Do you have on any socks, underwear, or clothing other than a hospital gown?—I think doctors and nurses take your clothes away so they will have the upper hand. I'm certain that it is not because they want to see our butts.
- Any jewelry or metal objects?—These could be used for escape tools.
- Any hairpieces, wigs, or prosthetics?—These would be great toys to play with while in the chamber, and I don't think they want you to have any fun.
- Any eyeglasses, hearing aids, books, magazines, newspaper or paper products?—They take these away so that they can be amused by watching you attempt to watch and listen to television on the tiny monitor without your glasses.
- Any cosmetics, hair products, shampoo, conditioner, or deodorant?—Again, I think doctors do this to make you feel inferior.
- Any battery-operated devices?—I'm not commenting on this one,

but I swear I get asked this question before every treatment.

- Any smoking materials?—Since you would have to be nuts to try to smoke in a 100 percent oxygen environment, I usually say "duh" when we come to this question.
- Any medication patches or any petroleum products?—Fortunately, Valium comes in tablet form, so I don't need any medication patches.
- Any nail polish less than twenty-four hours old?—Well, at least I don't have to get on my nail polish rant since I just need to plan all manicures and pedicures to fall on Friday afternoon or Saturday.
- Any dentures or loose dental work?—Now here I have a problem. I actually stopped the contraband interrogation at this point the other day to ask why no dentures. The nurse said it might be because if they spontaneously flew out of your mouth and landed between the gurney and the chamber wall, it could scratch the chamber when they pull you out. Then they would have to shut down the chamber until the scratch was buffed out. I call bull. Let me say that you can take my underwear, my eyeglasses, my hearing aid, and my entertainment, but you aren't taking my teeth! I don't wear dentures, but I'm drawing a line in the sand on this one.
- Any pain, chest pain, difficulty breathing?—These sound like legitimate questions. I'm not going to make jokes about them.
- Any changes in allergies since yesterday?—I just look at them. Seriously? I'm allergic to the same things I was allergic to yesterday. I promise.

Bonus Questions

Wednesday, April 16: Each nurse seems to have a bonus question she likes to ask that isn't on the original list. Some of the bonus questions have been:

- Any tissues?—I could actually see someone trying to take a tissue and forgetting about it. My mother-in-law always had one up her sleeve in case of a nasal emergency.
- Any Band-Aids?—Again, I could see a person forgetting they had a Band-Aid on.
- Any Neosporin?—Shame on someone for taking care of a wound! And you probably covered it with a Band-Aid, didn't you?
- Any gum or candy?—You can't blame someone from trying!

- Any hand sanitizer?—This was recently added to the list because of a germaphobic, compulsive hand washer—me! I always use hand sanitizer when I'm in a clinic or hospital, and in my defense, they did have hand sanitizer on the wall as I walked into the wound center. It resulted in my having to scrub my hands with Johnson's Baby Shampoo before my dive. On my last dive, I may point out that they have a soap dispenser in the changing room too, and it sure isn't filled with Johnson's Baby Shampoo (the only approved product I can use)!

Diabetic patients get to take orange juice in with them. I just get water (which I'm afraid to drink because there are no bathroom breaks). When the nurse walked by with the orange juice for my fellow diver on Friday, I asked for an Egg McMuffin. She got even by waving her iced cappuccino at me later in my dive and taking a big, satisfying slurp from the straw. It really was funny. I am glad my nurses have a sense of humor.

When I get tired of these repetitive questions, I think about what would happen if my husband were undergoing this treatment. I'm pretty sure he would cooperate the first day, but over time, he would ask them to provide scientific documentation with three sources to prove removing his underwear was necessary. And then the rules would get changed...and I would be on the sidelines doing my happy dance and giving him high fives.

And the Cupcake Goes To...

Friday, April 18: On my first day of hyperbaric treatments, the nurse explained what would happen during the procedure, completed a safety check, and then asked if I had any questions. Granted, I was doped up on Valium and was having difficulty connecting the dots, but I did have one big question in mind. "What happens if there is a fire?" I asked. She reassured me that they had a plan in place if there was a fire in the chamber. With wide eyes and the wheels of my brain turning, my mind went to horrible places, but I explained, "No. I meant what happens if there is a fire in the hospital while I'm diving?"

"Good question," the nurse responded. She explained that in the event of an actual hospital fire, the person in charge of the fire phone would call down to the hyperbaric unit immediately to let my nurses know where the fire was, because they knew that the HBO area and surgery would need extra time to evacuate. My nurse promised me that she would not leave me and would get me out of the chamber and to safety...whatever it took. She then told me no one had ever asked that question before.

Well, you can just call me a Boy Scout, because I always have a plan, and a plan B. Before I even left the waiting room, I had told Gene that if he heard the fire signal, I expected to see his face at the end of my diving chamber as he pushed me out of the hospital. "Pull the plug and don't worry about battery backup," I told him, "and wheel me to the freight elevator!" He laughed, but I was serious. If it takes twenty-two minutes to get me out of the chamber, I want a plan in place.

I spent a lot of time thinking about fire while I was in the HBO chamber. I stared at the fire hoods located on the wall next to my dive chamber and even asked if I could take one in with me. The answer was no, and I got another no to taking one of those fire blankets that firefighters use in with me, but it was worth a try. My plan B was to use my drinking water bottle as an emergency fire extinguisher. I even read the "Emergency Fire Evacuation" card attached to the dive chamber.

I managed to complete my twentieth dive yesterday and was given a giant cupcake from the nurses wishing me luck on my upcoming surgery. It was very sweet of them, and it touched me deeply. We all want to be good patients or even a special patient that the nurses look forward to caring for. I hope, despite my claustrophobia, deep need to use hand sanitizer, and quirky sense of humor, I was one of those patients.

Later in the day, I received a call from preadmissions to confirm my medical history, go over my medications, explain my surgery, and see if I had any questions. I sat with my preop folder in my lap and went through the first few questions when I hear a loud announcement in the background from where the nurse was calling. I swore it said there was a fire. The nurse paused, then continued with her questions. Once again, I heard the fire announcement. When the nurse paused a second time, I asked, "Do you need to evacuate? Because this can wait for another time." The nurse said no but she appreciated me asking.

When the announcement came a third time, she said, "Hold on a second while I see where the fire is located." She then told me that it was no problem because it was over in the cancer clinic.

When I got off the phone, I told Gene about the fire and how glad I was that it happened *after* my dive. I cannot imagine what I would do if I heard that announcement and saw the nurses scrambling while I was in the HBO chamber. Fortunately, it was well away from the HBO area, but a concerned look from the nurse would be about all it would take for me to start begging for release. My "good patient" plan would go by the wayside, and I would be squirting down the inside of the HBO chamber with my water bottle and fashioning a hood out of my blanket. Good thing they had already given me my cupcake!

Emergency Underwear

Sunday, May 18: Steven flew in to stay with me for ten days following my great escape from the hospital after reconstructive surgery. He was in charge of my pain medications and driving me to and from hyperbaric treatments and doctor's appointments. Since I was restricted from using both arms, he was literally my caretaker until Gene could get home from work.

The first week I was home, I was on round-the-clock pain medications. In my drug-induced haze, it would have been easy to make a mistake and take too many pain pills. So Danielle wrote up a schedule on a whiteboard for Steven to follow in drugging poor ol' mom. How many chances in a lifetime do you get that opportunity? I remember Steven's and my eyes growing large as Danielle wrote out the schedule. It seemed very complicated, and we both worried we wouldn't be able to follow the chart. As the days passed, the chart became invaluable. It was our road map for the day. Gene was in charge of nighttime medications—he didn't need a chart.

The second item necessary for survival during Steven's stay was the travel bag. This bag included a couple bottles of water, my pain medication, a movie to watch during hyperbaric treatment, a package of cheese crackers to eat on the way either to or from treatment (HBO treatments increase your metabolism, and you need to eat before and/or after), and a laptop for Steven to entertain himself.

Steven would always be standing at the door of the chamber with a wheelchair, a bottle of water, and some pain medication following my two-hour HBO treatments. He knew I would be hurting after lying on my back and moving onto the gurney. He was so considerate to make sure I could get some pain relief as soon as possible.

We had been traveling to and from town for about eight days when I glanced over to see Steven digging in the travel bag for my bottle of water. As he dug around, I saw a pair of my underwear peek out of the bag. That seemed odd. I didn't remember putting a pair of underwear in the bag, and I was certain it wasn't Steven's idea. Then it hit me that this was the same bag I had packed to take to the hospital. Since I was going to be there for a couple of days, I had packed a pretty, new pair of pajamas and a pair of underwear. Apparently, I had forgotten to take the underwear out when we changed the bag to our travel bag.

So for a week, Steven had been fishing through the bag and hadn't mentioned or questioned the underwear. I just could not resist. I looked at him and said, "You never know when you are going to need an emergency pair of underwear."

He didn't even blink before responding, "Isn't that the truth!" It hurt so badly to laugh, but it was worth it. A twenty-seven-year-old man should not have to see his mom's emergency underwear.

I finished my postop HBO treatments on Tuesday, and the nurses gave me another cupcake and told me that they would miss my smile and my sense of humor. They took excellent care of me while I was diving, but I was a little disappointed. I was hoping for a certificate that said I was a "Certified Dive Master." How many people do you know who have done thirty dives?

CHAPTER 10
FINAL RECONSTRUCTION

Getting Rid of Baggage

Thursday, April 24, 2014: I have been losing a lot of baggage lately. By that, I mean the faux-breast forms that come with mastectomy bras. Every time I purchase a camisole, bra, or sports bra intended for women who have had mastectomies, a faux-breast form comes included with the purchase—kind of like a bonus. I have a large variety of shapes and sizes of breast forms stored around my house.

Most of these forms are made of either foam rubber or quilt batting. I'm amused by what the manufacturers must think my other breast looks like, because these forms vary from egg shaped to triangular shaped. And let's face it: no one is fooled into believing these are real breasts. But I guess they are to get you by until you buy an expensive prosthetic or have reconstruction. And they are better than nothing—on most days.

The problem is, they don't want to stay put very well. Some bras have pockets, but the forms still try to escape out the side or ride up and show above the neckline of your shirt. Gene has a signal he gives me to tell me that my stuffing is poking out from the top of my shirt. Over time, I have become less self-conscious about just grabbing the form and shoving it down and back into my bra. But all that moving around causes some skin irritation. Most days, as soon as I get home, I grab the form and toss it somewhere. Then I have to remember to pick them up when we have visitors.

I don't know why, but lately the forms seem to have a mind of their own and pop out on occasion. While we were on vacation, my form kept trying to escape out of the top of my dress. Rather than be embarrassed, I told my family, "If something pops out while we are exiting the restaurant, just keep walking. I have plenty more at home." As we left the restaurant, we were in a single line weaving our way through the tables when I heard Steven say "Go, go, go, go, go!" And we all laughed hysterically.

It turns out that it is a good thing that I have decided to laugh at these awkward moments. I was downtown and parked in front of the courthouse last week, and I bent over to try to figure out the parking meter. (Notice that I skipped over why I was at the courthouse?) About that time, I felt something hit my foot, and I looked down to see my faux breast rolling down the grass, over the curb, and into the gutter. I stood up, glanced around to see if the stream of people walking by had noticed. Then I slid down the hill in my dress shoes to recover the form. I was very impressed that no one stopped to stare. I decided that it could have been more embarrassing if it happened while going to communion at church, but surely God wouldn't let that happen.

The final straw seems to have been at the DFW airport yesterday. The weather was warm, the faux breast was uncomfortable, and I had just had enough. So I pulled out the form and tossed it on the seat of the rental car. As it turns out, when you return a rental car, the attendant likes to make sure you take all of your belongings with you. Yes…it was still on the seat of the car. The nice gentleman returned my possession to me, and I smiled, thanked him, and walked to the nearest trash can and threw it away. I'm done with breast forms. Good thing my next reconstruction surgery is tomorrow. I will let you know how I decide to dispose of the other dozen (or eleven) breast forms.

Latissimus Dorsi Surgery

Monday, May 12: Before I get into my recovery stories, I thought I would do a quick explanation of the type of reconstruction surgery that I had. Because of the radiation damage to my skin and chest muscle area, the only option for reconstruction on my right side was a latissimus dorsi muscle flap transfer. In this five-hour surgery, an ellipse of skin and the latissimus dorsi muscle was tunneled under my arm from my upper back to my chest wall to create a reconstructed breast. A tissue expander was added to allow for expansion and an implant in approximately three months. (Yes, another surgery). A second surgeon was in the room to swap out my tissue expander on the left side for the permanent implant.

As I prepared for the surgery, both my plastic surgeon and my primary care provider explained to me that I would have severe limitations following surgery, as well as significant pain. My primary care provider held both my hands and looked me in the eye and said, "Kathy, you are going to have to take the pain medication." This got my attention. She knows that I hate pain pills and rarely take them even after surgery. Sometimes I don't even fill the prescription. So the fact that she was making such a point with me gave me some warning about what was to come.

I was fortunate to get my favorite seven o'clock surgery time slot. I love this early morning slot because you have to get up and going so early that you are looking forward to napping through surgery. Plus, there is less of a chance that you will get bumped to a later time. I was surprised that I wasn't as nervous as I was with my other surgeries. I suspect it was because they weren't looking for cancer; they were just working toward reconstruction.

After I dressed in my designer hospital gown, I was given some warm antibacterial wet wipes to wash everything from my neck to my knees. The nurse warned me that I would feel sticky afterward. She wasn't kidding. It felt like I had put soap on and had forgotten to rinse off. As I sat on the bed and flapped my elbows, trying to dry my underarms, the anesthesiologist came in to discuss my care during surgery. He spent quite a bit of time with me and assured me he would do all he could to reduce any postsurgery nausea.

About fifteen minutes prior to my surgery, my plastic surgeon came in with his arsenal of Sharpies. I stood naked with my arms spread straight out while he drew on my chest and back. It is a rather weird experience. I'm typically a modest person, so I felt uncomfortable even though I know he was going to see me without clothing in the OR. The surgeon marked the center line of my chest from my neck to my navel. Then he drew the underline and top line of my left breast and a similar line on the right. He drew more lines as I speculated on what they referenced, then he turned me around and started drawing on my back. When he sat back to study and admire his artwork, I said, "You missed a spot." He laughed and said that it is exactly what he would say in my position. I'm deciding he has a better sense of humor than I gave him credit for.

As soon as he left , the OR nurses came in and told Gene and Danielle to say their good-byes. I never like it when the nurses say this. It sounds very pessimistic! I always want to ask them if they know something I don't know. They gave me an injection that was supposed to calm me and make me not care. I looked the nurse in the eye and said, "I'm sorry for anything I say from this point forward," and she laughed. I heard Gene and Danielle laughing as they wheel me out of the room, and it made me smile.

I was wheeled to the OR, and I checked out the room. The operating table looked very different from other times that I'd been in the OR. There was a form for my face to rest in. I had been told I would spend a long time lying on my stomach as they harvested the muscle in my back, but seeing the table gave me some clue as to how they would accomplish this. I remarked to the nurse that the table didn't look very comfortable. The anesthesiologist looked me in the eye and told the nurse to give me the other half of the medication, and that is the last thing I remember. I pray that the second injection shut my mouth.

Finding "Worse"

Monday, May 12: I'm always fascinated by what people consider "very painful" or "the worst pain they have ever had." As I've gone through my battle with breast cancer and my share of procedures, I have found that I was able to tolerate the pain pretty well. To be honest, most of the time I lie about the pain. Generally, I lie because I think it will get me out of the hospital faster, which is always my number-one goal. So after my hysterectomy and after my mastectomies, I have rated my pain a three on the one-to-ten pain scale. My nurses look at me skeptically as I hunch over and make a break for the bathroom, because I know they won't let me go home until I can accomplish this task on my own. It is silly, really. No one believes me, yet I persist in my ruse so I can make my escape for home.

I had been warned that there would be significant pain associated with my surgery and recovery and that I would be in the hospital for three to four days. So, naturally, I planned in advance for my escape to be the morning of day three. In my mind, I'm tougher than the average patient, and I know that I will rest better at home than in the hospital. In retrospect, I probably should have read my own chapter "Pride Goeth before the Fall" before making plans. I suspect there are some good reasons for the doctor saying you can stay in the hospital four days postop.

I awake in postop recovery to the voice of a nurse asking if I am in pain. Maybe the beads of sweat on my forehead and my accelerated heart rate and breathing are visual clues. "Yes," I whisper. The nurse asks me to rate my pain. I barely know who I am and what just happened to me, much less remember the pain chart. I consider my response, and I don't remember "Holy shit!" being on the pain scale, so I say, "Five?" and look to see if this is an acceptable answer. I'm aware enough to know that is higher than I usually admit to, but I'm thinking it could possibly, in some way, be worse. As I start to wake up more, I find "worse."

The nurse comes back and asks if I'm still in pain. "Yes," I respond. She asks me to again rate the pain. I can't think clearly, and I look to her for the correct answer. "Give me a number," I'm thinking. I will agree to anything that gets me another pain medicine injection. I'm told that I need to take some deep breaths to increase my oxygen absorption. I give it a try and nearly cry out as my ribs and back hurt. I'm thinking breathing is highly overrated and if the nurse wants me to increase my oxygen, she should find another way to go about it. At some point I'm moved to my room and see Danielle and Gene waiting for me.

Once again, the nurse pokes, prods, checks vitals and sutures, and asks my pain level. "Three?" I say. Danielle does an intervention and explains my pain scale to the nurse. She then tells me the nurses aren't allowed to give me pain medicine unless I'm at least at a five. "Can I change my answer?" I ask. I spend the next twenty-four hours responding to the same question, remembering to say at least five when asked to rate my pain. I glare at the smiley-face pain chart in the room. I still think they need to have a "Holy shit!" category.

I'm told that I need to get out of bed and take a walk the evening of my surgery. Are they kidding? Danielle (also a nurse) looks me in the eye and says, "Mom, you don't have to go far." She knows I'm an overachiever and have planned my escape. I somehow make it to the door and back to the bed, whimpering the entire way. The nurse asks me what hurts. Is she serious? "My back and my ribs," I respond. She asks me why my back hurts. I quite simply do not have enough strength to respond.

Danielle says, "Read her chart!" God bless Danielle. I suspect the nurses read "breast reconstruction" and weren't familiar with my particular surgery since I was only the third patient to have this procedure done in this hospital. (Now that I am home, I will cut them some slack, but at the time, it was exasperating.)

The morning after surgery, I was scheduled to do a hyperbaric dive. As the time approached, I could not imagine how they were going to accomplish this with the amount of pain I was in. I was loaded into a wheelchair and taken down to the HBO center. Danielle came along and explained to the HBO nurses that I was in a lot of pain and couldn't move my right arm. The nurses in HBO were wonderful as they prepped me for my dive. All I can say is that I survived the dive and I found "worst yet" on the pain scale.

When I returned to my room, I was in so much pain I couldn't even speak. Danielle took one look at me and the tears in my eyes and told the nurse that I needed morphine, stat. Once again, God bless Danielle. After I had the injection, I rated the pain at a nine, but I meant twelve. Where is "worse" on the pain scale?

Fortunately, most of this is a hazy memory. I did make my escape on the morning of day three, but it wasn't my best idea. More on that later.

Making My Escape

Thursday, May 15: Prior to surgery, my surgeon told me I would need to stay in the hospital three to four days and then would need plenty of help when I returned home. So, naturally, I formed a plan to escape two days after surgery. I don't know why I come up with these plans, but I'm consistent.

When my surgeon came in the day after surgery, he informed me that he was leaving town for a meeting and explained who would be on call if I had any complications. He then asked when I wanted to go home. "Saturday morning," I promptly replied.

He looked at Gene and Danielle and said, "Okay, but if you aren't up to it, you can stay another day or two. Just let the nurses know." Score one for me. My plan was working.

On Saturday morning, I have a nurse who seems to be very experienced and who also seems skeptical of my plan. She checks my chart, and it says the doctor will release me if I choose to go home. It probably also says that I should stay at least another day. The nurse asks me some questions like "What are you thinking?" and "Are you sure?" She then starts this dialogue about how she sometimes wonders how patients are going to manage at home considering their condition. I know she is talking about me. But I have a plan, and I'm sticking to it. My chart probably didn't mention that we live thirty miles from the hospital.

I have a general surgeon and a nurse to take care of me, so I'm not particularly worried about being cared for. I am a little concerned about survival and the drive home, but a plan is a plan. Mostly I'm thinking that I will sleep better at home…if I survive the trip.

I plan my escape to happen thirty minutes after I take a dose of pain medication. I'm not a martyr, and I know I am going to need some pain relief to survive my great escape. The nurse loads me into the wheelchair, shaking her head the entire time. I get the feeling she expects me to come to my senses. I'm wheeled out to the parking lot, and Gene has had the forethought to bring a small step stool for me to use to get in the SUV. I whimper and perspire, but with help, I'm loaded into the vehicle.

There were two things I didn't plan for. I had forgotten about all the potholes and road construction between the hospital and my house. Cedar Rapids Roads Department estimates that there are ten thousand potholes that need to be filled after our harsh winter. It is like torture. Gene apologizes as we cross each bump, but I can't even respond. We do arrive home, though, and I have never been so happy to see a recliner. I take back every bad thing I have said about recliners in the past. Forget snazzy decor. "Every house should have a recliner and a shower chair" is my new motto.

The second thing I didn't plan for was a severe thunderstorm warning. The second day we were home, the sirens went off, and Gene said we needed to go to the basement. Was he kidding? I couldn't imagine doing stairs when I could barely walk. But we took them one step at a time as I carried an emergency supply of pain meds in case we were stuck down there for any length of time. When we got to the basement, Gene put me in an office chair with wheels and promised to wheel me wherever I needed to go. It was luxury! I told him that we might need to take that chair upstairs with us…in a month, when I had regained enough strength to climb the stairs. I may have to rethink the great escape in the future.

Wonder Woman Takes a Fall

Wednesday, May 28: I'm a terrible patient. I suspect it is because I have no patience for recovery. I want to be better now—immediately, not sometime in the future. I knew going into this surgery that the recovery would take quite a bit of time. In fact, prior to my surgery, my surgeon handed me six pages of postsurgery instructions that covered the next five years. My eyes grew wide as I flipped through the pages. But then I decided that these were instructions for the average patient, and I'm not average. I am Wonder Woman—or so I thought. I am now one month postop, and I can tell you that Wonder Woman took a fall. I'm feeling more like Humpty Dumpty waiting for all the king's horses and all the king's men to put me back together again.

The first week of postop is a blur. I would say that the pain medications did their job. I doubt that there is anything good that would come from remembering the pain and discomfort of that first week, other than as a reminder that I don't ever want to do this surgery again. I know that I was totally dependent on other people to help me. I lived on Cup-a-Soup because that was all I could lift with my left hand. A friend brought over some cheddar potato soup, and it was wonderful. But I couldn't get the potatoes out of the bottom of the cup because I could only use one arm and only lift it so high. I just stared at the potatoes and sighed.

One thing I do remember from the first week was the bizarre dreams I would have while on the pain medications. One afternoon, I was staring at Gene and Steven suspiciously, certain that I should be mad at them. It took me some time to sort through what was real and what was a dream. That was the day I decided to quit taking prescription pain medication.

I was able to ditch the wheelchair after the first week postop and make it down to the hyperbaric department under my own steam. I also started using my left arm more and more. I was able to dress myself but still couldn't lift anything heavier than a paperback book. The right arm needed to remain at my side until week four. As the four Jackson-Pratt (JP) drains were removed, I became more comfortable. My brother refers to JP drains as grenades, which makes me laugh. I practically needed a tool belt to hold four drains across my stomach. You can imagine the fashion difficulties.

After the second week, each day showed vast improvements, and I ditched the restrictions for the left arm. Seriously, how long can a person go without using either arm? So I told my left arm to suck it up and started using it. I felt more comfortable and could walk farther every day. My restrictions included no twisting or lifting. At this point I became very good at picking things up with my toes. I started to use the computer by typing left handed. Dinner involved takeout or anything located on the middle three shelves of the pantry. My nurses were full of praise on how fast I was improving, but it has been very difficult.

And this is the point where I have started losing my mind. At one month, I have grown tired of recovery and glare at the postop instructions each time I pass them. I have found that the restrictions must have some scientific/medical basis, because when you ignore them, you pay for it. When Gene comes home and can see that I'm hurting, he asks, "What did you do today?" Why would he ask that? My look of innocence is lost on him as I shake out a couple ibuprofen from the bottle.

I know that my recovery is on schedule and that it will take time, but I want to be Wonder Woman, not Humpty Dumpty.

Nipple Tattoos

Saturday, June 13: Ah, where to start? I have been waiting for my surgeon to bring up this topic, and he finally mentioned it this week. I had asked him if he felt that he could finish my reconstruction all in one single surgery, when he replies, "That should be possible unless you want to do nipple tattoos." Now he has my undivided attention.

I pipe up with the line I have been saving for months: "Oh no. I plan to use stickers." He doesn't even blink or pause. Hmm. Then he explains that yes, there are plenty of stickers available, but I should at least consider the tattoos.

Well, hold the bus right here. I had no idea there were real nipple (areola) stickers available. My plan was to go to the dollar store and pick up a couple of sticker sheets with silly shapes or characters and surprise Gene now and then. My girlfriends are already entertaining me by dropping sheets of stickers in the mail. I make a mental note to check out the nipple stickers when I get home.

My surgeon explains that he attended a recent conference where one of the topics was nipple tattooing. I swear, I am keeping my mouth shut because I am too entertained to speak. But I'm thinking that if I were attending a conference, and that topic was on the agenda, I would have a front-row seat. "You would think that the last place you might want to go for nipple tattoos would be a tattoo shop," he says, "but it turns out that tattoo artists do a far more realistic job of nipple tattooing than many medical professionals."

My doctor explains that medical tattoos tend to be flat and single-dimensional, where tattoo artists go for more of a 3-D effect. He gives me the name of a nipple-tattoo artist who is nationally known for his work (everybody has to be good at something!) and tells me to go home and check out his website before I make a decision. This is one homework assignment that I can't wait to start!

So last night, I fire up my laptop while Gene and I are watching television. I tap away and Google the tattoo artist's name and immediately find his website. Sure enough, he comes up as the number-one nipple-tattoo artist on Google. As soon as I get to his website, my security settings prevent me from seeing the images. Without looking up, I ask Gene, "How do I change my security settings so I can look at nipple tattoos?" All I hear is silence. After a few moments, I look up, and he is just staring at me. I try to keep a straight face, but seriously, this is too much fun. Gene has been doing breast cancer surgery for twenty-five years, so he knows a trap when he hears one. He isn't going to comment.

I figure out how to crack my security myself, and sure enough, there are dozens of images of nipple tattoos. I have to stop for a moment to admire the work because this guy is really, really good at his job. There are a variety of sizes and colors, and even some photos of men who have had mastectomies and nipple tattoos. I'm cruising along the photos when I have to stop in my tracks. There is a photo of a nipple tattoo with a piercing. My mouth opens. Holy cow, I need to get out more. After the initial shock, I laugh and think, "Good for you." After all the surgeries, treatments, reconstruction, and all it takes to beat breast cancer, I applaud someone who has the imagination and sense of humor to have an artificial piercing added to her nipple tattoo.

Since I'm doing homework, I decide to find out what is available in nipple stickers. Once again, I wonder what people did for entertainment before the Internet. I find that there are many types of stickers: rub-on temporary nipple tattoos, gel stickers, bumper stickers, you can even customize your stickers. I did not click on the link that advertised "cheap nipple stickers." I think if you are going to go to the trouble of buying nipple stickers, you don't want to go cheap and can spring for the extra dollar or two.

Tattoos vs. stickers—I would like to say the jury is still out, but I'm pretty sure I won't be getting tattoos. However, I reserve the right to change my mind, and if I do, I'm traveling the two thousand miles to check out this nationally known nipple-tattoo artist—and I'm either taking my best friend, Tess, or my sister, Tammy, with me for the entertainment value. I promise not to take my son Steven, who has PTSD after the emergency underwear event. I wonder if the travel expense would be covered by insurance.

Expansions

Wednesday, August 6: I had another tissue expansion done last week, and I winced as the doctor filled my expander with saline. It wasn't because the procedure was particularly uncomfortable or painful. I winced because I was pretty sure the water balloon under my skin was going to burst and put my eye out. The doctor casually chatted with my husband as I held my breath. When the nurse asked if I was okay, the doctor looked at my expression and asked if I was in pain. "No, but is my breast supposed to be up at my collarbone?" I ask.

We had a brief discussion about whether the expander had rotated and now was sitting up and down, rather than side to side. The doctor told me not to worry about it at this point because he was just trying to create space for the permanent implant. The shift was simply because my radiated skin was not expanding, so the expander had no place to go but up. He promised that he can fix it at surgery.

I trust that my doctor can make my chest look better after my final surgery next month, but in the meantime I have a predicament. I have a breast on my collarbone. Sort of like Quasimodo in reverse. As we walked out of the doctor's office, I said to Gene, "Just great! I have a boob on my shoulder. Have you ever seen someone walking around with a boob poking out of the top of her shirt?"

Gene didn't pause before saying, "No comment." This made me laugh. Some women work hard to make their breasts visible, so I should look at this as a free benefit of cancer! Too bad it is all one sided.

Rehab

Sunday, August 10: I passed the three-month-postop mark and started physical therapy to regain strength and range of motion in my chest, back, shoulders, and core. Matt is my new personal trainer. He is one of the perks that come with being a cancer patient. His services are covered by a community grant, so no deductibles, no copays, no hassle. As I walked into the gym, Matt gave me the once-over, and I knew immediately what he was thinking: "She has a *lot* of potential!"

Matt put me through a series of exercises to test my balance, my strength, and my attention span. When he completed the evaluation, he declared me "better than average." I was feeling pretty good about this until I remembered that I am considered young for a breast cancer patient, so average would be someone in her sixties. Now I'm not sure how I ranked.

I left physical therapy with three sheets of exercises to work on daily at home. Our goal is to get my range of motion and strength back to normal before my last surgery next month. When Matt told me that at that point, we would start back at square one, it was a bit discouraging. But he promised that rehab after the last surgery will go much quicker.

Before I left the gym, Matt cautioned me to start slowly and work my way up to the recommended number of sets and repetitions. I tend to be an overachiever and knew I would ignore his caution at the first opportunity. As soon as I got home, I pulled my daughter's old gymnastics mat out to do the floor exercises on. I circled it a couple times, wondering when the floor became so far away. I was pretty sure I could successfully get down on the mat but not so certain I could get back up.

Fully committed to starting my rehabilitation, I managed to get down on the mat without falling. I sat for a few minutes to get comfortable, when along came our new dog, Luci. Suddenly, I had ninety pounds of German shepherd in my lap demanding a belly rub. She thinks physical therapy is great! We have had her only a month, and this was the first time she had ever seen me on the floor, so she was taking advantage of it. I get partial credit for shoving ninety pounds of enthusiasm off my lap.

As I worked through the exercises, I felt betrayed by my body. I recognized most of the exercises as things I have done all my life—lie on the floor on your back and extend your hands above your head while pointing your toes—only my body wouldn't do those things. In one exercise where you lie on your back, bend one knee, and cross it over your body, nothing happened on the right side. How could that be? The left side worked. I know the doctor moved a muscle from my back to my chest, but surely the muscle should still work. I groaned, I grunted, but that knee was not going over my body. I did get a well-deserved lick from Luci for my efforts.

I finished the floor exercises and rolled over to try to stand up. Luci thought this was great fun. I, on the other hand, was dizzy and nauseated. I managed to crawl over to the bed and heave myself up. As I sat taking deep breaths and praying that the room would quit spinning, I heard Matt's voice in my head telling me to start slowly. Well, I have only a month to recover before my next surgery, so my body is just going to have to suck it up and get over it.

When Gene got home that evening, he asked how rehab went. I told him that it made me dizzy and nauseated and that everything hurt. He replied that he had worked with rehab all of his surgical career and never once had he heard of that as a goal of rehabilitation. I would have punched him in the arm if I could have lifted my own arm. I did consider siccing Luci on him.

My neck hurts, I'm walking with a slight limp from pulling a calf muscle, and my shoulder is throbbing. I am determined to get back to normal, but I may have to learn moderation. I also plan to move the mat closer to the bed so it is easier to get up.

The Finish Line

Wednesday, September 17: My final reconstruction surgery is scheduled for Friday, and I'm rather looking forward to it. It is as though I can see the finish line and can't wait to cross it. I have crossed off so many goals and milestones in my journey with cancer, but the big goal—finishing—has always been off the horizon.

Gene and I had a mini-celebration last night and blew up some tomatoes from the garden, some old eggs, and my favorite target: a stale can of biscuits. I laughed so hard when Gene shot the can and biscuit dough started spurting out in a stream. I laughed even harder this morning when I saw the empty can at the edge of the forest. It appears that raccoons had a feast on pieces of tomato, broken eggs, and biscuit dough. They were rude enough to leave the can behind.

Stage two of reconstruction will include replacing the temporary tissue expander with my permanent implant, leveling my breasts, some final tweaks, and my favorite—a fat transplant. I kid you not. All these years I have been offering to be a donor for a fat transplant, thinking it was a made-up procedure, and it turns out there really is such a thing. Well, sign me up.

The fat transplant (fat grafting) involves reverse liposuction, as I like to call it. The doctor will take fat from someplace on my body where I have spare fat. (Are they kidding? Take your pick of location!) The doctor managed to make this statement without adding any additional comment about so many possibilities. He will then inject the fat above my implant to make the breast look a bit more normal. I think this is one of those cases where having some extra weight on board is an advantage. As I told my mom this morning, "I think fat people have an easier time with cancer than skinny people. We have more reserves."

The leveling of my breasts is due to skin damage from radiation. The right-side skin has not stretched like the doctor was hoping it would. So we need to raise the left breast so that they are level and plumb. (I just added that last part for fun.) I have been wearing shirts with prints to disguise the imbalance for several months, so it will be nice to have my clothes fit better in the future. But what will make me "unique" once everything is balanced?

The surgery is scheduled to take three hours, and I'm sad to say that preparing for surgery is becoming routine now. The laundry is done, the plants have been pruned, my desk is clean, and my calendar has been cleared. My friend Joanne is taking care of Luci Dog and house-sitting. I have a week's worth of meals prepared and in the freezer, but Gene promises he has the pizza place on speed dial in case of emergency.

Tess is coming to town for the surgery and for entertainment. She thinks I'm funny after anesthesia and doesn't want to miss anything. I explained to her that if all goes well and my surgery starts on time, I might possibly be able to go home on Friday. She just laughed and said she was coming anyway. She finds my unrealistic goals amusing. I should have a short two-week recovery, then arm and shoulder rehab again. I'm becoming a professional at rehabilitating a shoulder. My favorite exercise is to reorganize the shelves in my pantry to see how high I can stretch my arm. Maybe that should be my next profession: Shoulder Rehab Ltd.—*We will have you back to organizing your pantry in no time!*

I do have plans for a spectacular grand finale at the end of the month—two years to the date of my diagnosis. My sister and brother-in-law will be here visiting from Texas. I don't want to ruin the surprise, but the grand finale involves a lot of pumpkins, a lot of Tannerite, and a lot of bra-stuffing material!

Beware of the Blue-Light Special

Saturday, October 4: I remember shopping with my mother in K-Mart when I was a child and hearing the announcement, "Attention, K-Mart shoppers. We have a blue-light special on aisle four," and we would rush over to see what the incredible special was. Later, when we returned home, we would wonder what we were going to do with twelve various colors of thread that we had picked up for the incredible, one-time price of $3.99! The deal sounded so good that you didn't take the time to think it through.

That's kind of how I felt after surgery. As mentioned, my surgeon told me that while he was doing the finishing touches on my breast reconstruction, he could liposuction some "extra" fat and place it around my implant for a more natural look. Sort of a fat transplant. Silly me. I heard "liposuction" and envisioned a quick way to move some fat from where I didn't want it to where I did want it and didn't think through the procedure. It turns out liposuction sucks! Both figuratively and literally.

Once again, the OR nurse injected Versed into my IV as he wheeled me out of my preop room. I'm getting pretty good at spotting the Versed and making my advance apologies quickly. My nurse asked me if it made me talkative. "No," I replied, "it makes me reorganize the OR and tell you how to do your job more efficiently." He laughed, and we began discussing the recent remodel of the OR floor as he wheeled me through the halls. The last thing I remember saying was, "You know, they should have increased the size of the holding rooms a few inches while they were at it." I'm sure he was laughing as he continued to wheel me to my OR, and I'm also pretty sure that I kept organizing things as we went.

When I woke in recovery, I looked at my nurse and said, "I need to tell you something," only I couldn't remember what I needed to tell her. It turns out that I told her Gene was a doctor and Danielle was in charge of the emergency room. (Danielle thought that was pretty funny.) I just know that my brain was very scrambled, and I was trying to put the pieces together. When asked to rate my pain, I said, "I don't know. Give me a number." These kind of test questions when you first wake up are just too hard and don't get easier with each surgery.

As I became clearer headed, the pain started setting in, and I took inventory of what hurt. I felt like I was being strangled by a boa constrictor as I shifted and whimpered. Later I would learn that I was wrapped in two mile-long Ace wraps from below my armpits to my lower hips. I looked like a mummy. There is something claustrophobic about being wrapped so tightly, especially when you know you have to leave the compression in place for a couple weeks. The doctor told Gene that if the lower wrap bothered me too much, I could remove it. I lasted two days…maybe.

While I expected the pain below my implants and under my arms, I was surprised at how uncomfortable my abdomen was. Who knew fat could hurt? Seriously, I never even gave it a thought before surgery. I can tell you now that liposuction hurts…a lot. Who would voluntarily sign up for that? I have two small incisions in my lower belly, and two weeks later, I am bruised black, blue, and green across my entire abdomen. It is still tender. The swelling is still going down, so the jury is out on whether I will notice a difference/reduction in belly fat. I can say that the fat transplant was effective in giving a more normal appearance to my bustline, except that I'm also black and blue on my chest and shoulder as well. I look like someone who has either been in a car accident or a boxing match.

There are times you lose a lot of your dignity when you go through breast cancer treatment. One of these moments occurred when I had to go to the bathroom before being released from the hospital. I sat up in bed and groaned as I swung my legs over the side of the bed just a couple hours after surgery. Danielle and my nurse helped walk me to the bathroom, and when we got there, we all realized my dilemma at the same time. I was wrapped in an Ace wrap clear down to my lower hips. "Um, how do I do this?" I asked. There was no quick way to get me out of the Ace wrap, and I wasn't sure what was under it. The nurse said, "Hold on, I'm going to take a quick peek," and she did. "You're clear," she said. If I hadn't needed to go to the bathroom so badly, I would have been embarrassed. Sometimes you just have to let someone help you.

I will say that my surgeon did a beautiful job in removing the extra tissue under my arms, and when I quit hurting, I think I will be happy with the result. Because of radiation damage, my breasts will never fool anyone who sees them into thinking they are my natural breasts, but I wasn't planning any topless beaches in my future anyway. I have so many scars that I look like a patchwork quilt. My goal was to have a more normal appearance when fully clothed. And as I told Gene, I have so many numbered parts (implants) that I will be easy to identify if they find me buried in a shallow grave in the woods. "Good to know," was his reply.

The Empathy Factor

Friday, September 26: I have read that dogs have the uncanny ability to sense their owners' emotions and needs. There was even a recent news story about one dog's ability to predict seizures in its owner. I am certain that our last dog, Dolly Dog, knew that I was unwell, and she slept next to the sofa and kept watch as I recovered from chemo. She held on and lay by my side as long as she could but died last fall. Now we have Luci Dog, and she is another story entirely.

Since Luci recently graduated from dog training school, I felt somewhat confident that I would be able to get in the door on my return from the hospital without getting mowed down. Just to be sure, Gene got me into the house and into the recliner before releasing the beast. Luci was excited to see me but on her way over was distracted by her ball, and she stopped to pick it up and drop it in my lap. I tried not to cringe as she barreled toward me. Gene took her for a quick walk and bribed her with her favorite treat (baby carrots) on his return just to keep her distracted. We call carrots "motivators" since she will follow you anywhere and try out all her tricks just to get one.

Gene did his best to keep her distracted the first couple of days home, but Luci requires a certain amount of petting from each of us each day, and she was not going to let me off the hook. Her ninety pounds of insistence as she shoved her nose under my elbow and threw my arm in the air was a less than subtle reminder that she was being neglected. I showed her my doctor's orders that clearly stated that I could not move my arm that much for four weeks, but she didn't care. Nor did she care that I was recovering. She loves Gene the most and thinks of him as her personal play toy, but she has come to expect extra walks during the day with just the two of us.

Luci's point was that I had adopted her and agreed to take care of her. That care requires multiple walks, no less than seven petting episodes of varying duration, food and water, and at least four baby carrots per day. So suck it up, buttercup, let's go for a walk. I managed to walk Luci three times today, with a handy stash of motivators (carrots) in my pocket to ensure cooperation from all those involved. I could see the wheels turning as she tried to decide between chasing a squirrel into the woods and her odds of getting a carrot afterward. "Don't make me come after you," I said to her. "I like carrots too, and I will eat that carrot right in front of you if you make me chase you." My doctor says that walking is good for me. I'm thinking about loaning him Luci for a day.

Getting Good Help

Thursday, October 16: Tomorrow marks my last day of restrictions from my last surgery. I'm so excited. I will be able to extend my arms beyond the strike zone! For the past four weeks, I have been asked not to lift anything heavier than a gallon of milk or raise or extend my right arm beyond ninety degrees. So basically, anything outside of the baseball strike zone has been outside of my reach. I have found two ways to get around the restrictions: get creative and find good help.

There are a couple of tools that are beneficial when you have limited reach—a back scratcher, a pair of cooking tongs, toes, a grabber tool, and a tongue. I have used the back scratcher to help pull my compression bra off when Gene isn't home and to scratch the hard-to-reach areas. The tongs and grabber tool (like advertised on TV for old people to get cans off of high shelves) are extremely useful in extending my reach to get the coffee filters off the top shelf of the pantry. I'm getting good at catching things that I can just wriggle off of a high shelf with one of my tools. I have used my toes to pick up anything that dropped to the floor. And finally, my tongue. When I'm having trouble reaching something, I tend to bite the point of my tongue as I struggle to extend my reach yet stay within my restrictions. Gene says, "You know that really doesn't help, don't you? Would you like me to help you?" It is like through sheer willpower I can extend my reach just a bit more.

Getting good help is probably the key to recovery after surgery. I have been so fortunate to have friends and family step in and help me after my surgeries. It is a humbling experience for me, and I hope to help others in the future to pay back the debt I have accumulated. The best part of having good help is the entertainment factor.

Tess decided to come stay with us for a few days after my surgery. Tess is always great entertainment, and the chance to have her company for two days was like getting a treat after going to the dentist. The first day she stayed with me, I mostly slept. I woke up at one point and saw Tess asleep in a matching recliner, and I smiled. I thought, "Only a family member or very good friend could spend a beautiful day napping in a recliner beside me." It was so peaceful. Tess kept my water glass filled, handed me my pain meds, helped me out of my chair, and helped Gene prepare dinner. We talked and told stories and laughed.

At dinner, she looked over and said, "Okay, girlfriend. Tomorrow we are getting into the shower together and washing your hair!" I snuck a glance at Gene, who was sitting back in his chair with a grin on his face, anticipating my reply.

I paused a beat and replied, "Great. Another new experience for my blog." I tried to put some enthusiasm into the statement, but the mental images going through my head were holding me back.

I will admit, I cheated. Nothing like fear of humiliation to motivate a person. I got up early and had Gene help me shower. We could not wash my hair in the shower due to all of my dressings, but I was clean and felt better. I am very modest, and the thought of someone other than Gene seeing me without my clothes on caused a lot of anxiety. In fact, I like to think that the OR staff and surgeon have seen only the incision area of my body. I had enough tubes and tape after surgery to know better, but I try not to think about how exposed I was.

Tess just laughed when I told her that I had already showered, and said, "But I wanted to do your hair." So we compromised, and I leaned over the laundry room sink as she washed and conditioned my hair. I then sat in a chair in my bathroom as she dried and styled my hair, teaching me how to "confuse my hair" as she dried it—a trick she uses to relax some of the curl. I should mention that Tess is an attorney, not a hairstylist. She also happens to be part owner of a chain of hair salons, so this may have convinced her that she has some hair-styling expertise. While she may not be a trained stylist, she had two working arms and time on her hands, so I was willing to let her have her way with me. Tess instructed me on various curl-relaxing products (which I suspect can be purchased only at her chain of salons) and sprayed and squirted half a pound of product in my hair. Honestly, I wasn't listening. I was simply enjoying the luxury of having my hair washed and styled and feeling happy that she didn't see me naked. Tess is good help.

My next helper is my friend Becky. I had planned to try to drive myself to my one-week follow-up appointment so that I didn't have to inconvenience any of my friends. As I got closer to the appointment, I realized that it would not be safe for me to make the thirty-mile trip on my own. Sometimes I wonder what doctors are thinking when they schedule a one-week follow-up. Becky stepped in and offered to drive an hour each way to pick me up and take me to my appointment. Becky has been fabulous at taking me or meeting me at these surgery follow-up appointments.

I can't undress myself without help at this point. Becky and the nurse helped unwrap the mile-long Ace wrap that binds my chest, remove the gauze, and get me into a gown. It was exhausting, but we laughed as I turned in circles and they gathered the Ace wrap into a pile. Becky has already seen my bare chest because she has escorted me to several of these appointments. I try not to let it bother me. I know with certainty that Becky will not judge me or talk to others about what I look like without my shirt on, so that comforts me. Becky is good help.

The surgeon came in to free me from my many attachments. He removed sutures, the drain, Steri-Strips, gauze, and foam—all sorts of things. If you have ever had a JP drain, you will understand when I say my doctor is *good* help! Getting the drain out was worth whatever the charge was. The doctor leaned back and inspected his work. I am very swollen and black and blue, but I can already tell that the work he did under my arms is fabulous, and I told him so. He seemed pleased. The doctor told me that this was a hard procedure and he was actually quite uncomfortable while he was doing it. I didn't pause a beat before replying sympathetically, "Ohhh, I'm so sorry you were uncomfortable during my surgery."

The doctor and nurse chuckled, and he said, "I get it." I think he is becoming used to my sarcasm.

My sister and brother-in-law came for a weeklong visit a week after my surgery. They cooked and entertained me. Best of all, they entertained Luci Dog. Luci is not good help. She doesn't care that I have had surgery. She wants her morning, noon, and afternoon walks regardless of how slowly I am moving or how much discomfort I am feeling. She will stand and look at whatever I have dropped on the floor and refuse to pick it up for me. Or worse yet, if she does pick it up, she will haul it off to some place where I will never find it. She has perfected playing fetch with me by rolling her ball to hit my feet. When I kick or nudge the ball, she chases it and brings it back, and the game starts all over again. She is not service-dog material.

Each day showed significant improvement and led toward my three-week checkup. I drove my own darn self to my appointment and took pleasure in it. When my nurse met me in the reception area, she said, "You look so good! Where's your entourage?"

To which I responded, "I ran out of friends," and we laughed.

I am doing well and looking forward to life without restrictions. I have been blessed to have good help.

Big Bang!

Thursday, November 6: My sister and brother-in-law came to visit, supposedly to celebrate the end of reconstruction. Personally, I think they just wanted to blow some things up. After three surgeries, twelve weeks of restrictions, seven JP drains, and enough scars to form a patchwork quilt, I was finally done with reconstruction, and I wanted to go out with a big bang. We picked a beautiful fall day to celebrate the finish line. With Tannerite, breast forms, pumpkins, and weapons in hand, we went out to a field to cause some carnage.

After gathering all of my temporary breast forms, we had a serious discussion on how we were going to blow them up. The guys were trying to be tactful and respectful, but my sister and I were having none of it. My first idea was to get a piece of cardboard and glue all the forms on it, creating one giant boob. I even planned to paint the center form red to make a nipple. But logistics and gravity were against me, so on to plan B. Gene came up with the idea of putting the forms in a giant, clear pork-rind container. Oddly enough, you can't buy such large containers of pork rinds in Iowa (the Pork State) but have to import them from Texas. There was something funny about stuffing faux boobs into a pork-rind container. At this point, there was a lengthy discussion about the process and what gun to use. We let the boys work it out.

Gene placed the container on a stump, and we all put our earplugs in. Tammy and I got our cameras ready and prepared to document the explosion. Gene took one shot, and boom! Breast forms and the lid when flying as we all held our sides and laughed.

We finished off the day by blowing up pumpkins, which has become symbolic of my progress. So many people have asked, "Why are you blowing up pumpkins?" I have two responses to that question. First of all, because it is fun! You can't help but laugh when a pumpkin explodes and pieces fly everywhere. And the other reason is that I needed something to mark the progress through each stage of this journey called breast cancer. I also knew that whatever symbol I used, I wanted it to be funny.

I think that my dream finale would have been to have a pumpkin patch drop a truck full of pumpkins at the house and have all my friends bring lawn chairs and sit and cheer as we blew them up in one big explosion. Maybe we will save this for my three-year anniversary!

Good Enough

Monday, November 17: I had my two-month follow-up appointment with my plastic surgeon last week and got my topless photos taken for my chart once again. When the doctor said he wanted to take another set of photos, I sighed and just continued to sit on the table. The nurse started laughing and said, "He wants photos of you, not me!" I laughed. I don't know what I was thinking. I'm pretty sure he would win the stalemate if I just continued to sit there, but I just hate knowing those photos are out there.

The surgeon talked about some minor tweaks that could be made to enhance my new breasts' appearance, but I told the doctor that I felt we had reached "good enough." Sometimes I don't think we know when to stop, but I have maxed out my attention span for reconstruction. Sure, we could add some more fat grafting, raise one side to be more level with the other side, or even add nipple tattoos, or any of a number of other tweaks.

But let's face it: I'm never going to walk on a topless beach and fool anyone into thinking these breasts are real/natural. And honestly, if I were shipwrecked on a deserted island, I would not go topless until I simply ran out of clothing. My best bet would be to be shipwrecked with my daughter, Danielle, who travels with more clothing than anyone I know. When you ask her about it, she claims it is in case no one else's luggage shows up. She will have enough for everyone to have something to wear.

So I am calling "good enough," and I feel happy with the final result. I can walk into a room without slouching and feel confident that I have a natural appearance. I am done, done, done, done, done with reconstruction!

CHAPTER 11
SURVIVING

Retrospect

Monday, December 1, 2014: Now that treatment and reconstruction are over, I find myself with time to look back and analyze a few things. It was important to me to write about my feelings and thoughts while going through treatment, but there were some things that were just too difficult to share at the time. As I talked with Tess today, we each shared how we were feeling as I was diagnosed with cancer, our fears, and how those fears changed and were resolved in the first few months.

I remember living with fear for the first month. It could have been paralyzing except that I was so busy going from appointment to appointment and processing information and medical terms that I didn't have the choice to be paralyzed. I wrestled with wondering if this was all the time that I had. Would I survive surgery? Would chemo kill me? What was my survival chance? How would I possibly tell my children? It was all-consuming.

Tess, on the other hand, was struggling to be positive and supportive yet worried that the disease would kill me. She shared that she was so worried at first that I wouldn't survive this. And then once she decided I was going to survive, she wondered how bad the treatment would be for me and how she could help me get from point A to point B. She became the person I could call on my drive to treatment who would somehow acknowledge that "this sucked" and then make me laugh as I was walking into the building.

I remember the day I had to call my children to tell them I had cancer. I didn't want to tell them while they were at work. They were still recovering from the call about the death of my father just two weeks earlier. How on earth could I drop more weight on their shoulders? How could I reassure them?

I remember each call distinctly. I managed not to cry when I spoke to each of my children. I wanted to be calm and reassuring, to be Mom, but my heart was breaking. I tried to say all the right words, but it was exhausting. I sobbed after each phone call. I know I could have let Gene make the calls, but I felt they would be more reassured if they spoke to me. I encouraged them to call Gene if they had any questions. I remember the sweetest words from my twenty-six-year-old son: "I love you, Mama."

Letting the rest of my family know was equally difficult. We had just buried my father. We were already so sad. I could not imagine adding this burden to their hearts. Then I had to notify close friends. Once again, Tess stepped forward to help make calls. I was out of energy. I think it was at this point that I realized I could not do this alone. I was going to need help.

I waited to notify my clients until last. It was one of the most difficult e-mails I have ever written. As a small-business owner, I have worked so hard to build a business, and I was afraid that I was about to lose that business. My son offered to step up and manage the business for me for the next year. I was incredibly grateful and appreciative. Even though I offered to help my clients find other website designers, they all opted to stay with us. I have wonderful clients.

The next big hurdle was asking Gene what my survival chances were. It had to be Gene who I asked. I hated to put him in this position—being my physician as well as my husband—but I knew I wouldn't be able to get the words out at the doctor's office. It broke my heart that I might be putting him in the position of telling me terrible news, and I didn't want to cry when I asked him. I knew he would be honest.

Waiting for surgery and wondering how I would feel emotionally afterward was awful. But I have to say that a huge weight was lifted off my shoulders once the mastectomy was over. It was a big relief to have the cancer out of me. I didn't have the emotional reaction over losing a breast that some people have. I was just grateful that the cancer was removed.

My next fear was that chemo would kill me. It was several weeks after I started chemo before I voiced this concern to Gene. He was shocked. He explained that there was no way the doctor would let chemo kill me. If it got to the point that I couldn't tolerate the treatment, they would stop treatment. He explained that the cancer was most likely gone and chemo was just to improve my chances of not having a recurrence. So there was no way the doctors would risk my death on something that was just increasing my survival rate.

This was one of many conversations we had where Gene saw cancer from a patient's perspective and how easily these misconceptions came about. I didn't often share these concerns with my doctors. I should have. I might have had an easier time of it. I remember one conversation with my doctor when she said, "I can't help you if you don't talk to me." But I wanted to appear strong. I wanted to be an easy patient.

In retrospect, my treatment wasn't as bad as I feared it would be. It wasn't easy. Sometimes it was incredibly difficult, and I don't want to ever go through it again. But many of the things that I feared were baseless or didn't happen. Other things were more difficult than I expected. This is a journey of ups and downs.

My Mother

I have had a lot of support from family and friends during this journey through breast cancer, and one of my strongest supporters has been my mother. She got on a plane all by herself after not flying for fifteen years in order to be here for my surgery. She sat up in the early hours of the morning and talked with me when I couldn't sleep. She flew in to help me (and watch me sleep) during the last week of phase two of chemo. She has spent hours and hours on the phone talking with me and ended each call with the assurance that I could call her and talk to her about anything.

But the thing that gets to me is when she tells me how proud she is of how I have handled myself throughout this journey. It chokes me up. Each time she says this, I want to tell her that I learned strength from her. As a child, teenager, and adult, I have known that I could ask her anything—I could tell her things that I wasn't proud of, my fears, or my dreams, and she would be a safe haven. She has counseled me my entire life. She is the one who taught me to work calmly through an emergency and fall apart later. She taught me grace, kindness to others, and how to listen. And she can deliver a punch line better than any comedian.

I suspect it must be horrible to watch your child go through cancer, and to have to do this just weeks after losing your husband of fifty-five years would be enough to break anyone. But my mother has shown such strength and compassion. We have learned about cancer and the treatment process together. We have laughed at the indignities of diagnosis and treatment and my irreverence. We have talked about life and the possibility of death. She was in the room when I looked at my scar for the first time and I said, "I can live with that," and meant it. And she has let me cry when I needed to and has understood when I asked, "When will I feel safe again?"

And yet my mom says she is proud of me. Look in the mirror, Mom.

Chance of Cure (Survival Rate)

I find myself struggling with this subject. Not because the news is bad but because I want to present the information fairly and accurately. One of the things that I have found interesting through this journey is the philosophical differences between specialists and how they treat the question of survival. I ask my readers to recognize that this is my interpretation of my specific diagnosis and encourage you to talk with your physicians about your specific prognosis.

Whenever a friend or family member is diagnosed with cancer, I ask Gene what his or her chance of survival is. I usually ask him about a specific type of cancer and give him the information I have been told, then ask about survival. He is always honest with me. He tells me when he isn't familiar with a specific disease or doesn't have enough information. He tells me what the variables are, and then gives me the statistics. So when the time came, I knew I could ask Gene what my chance of survival was. I know this was unfair to him, and I hated to put him in the position of possibly telling me bad news. But I trust him completely.

Like most patients, I suspect, I wanted to know what my chance of survival was almost immediately. I kept waiting for one of my physicians to give me the information. None did. A couple of times, I almost asked the doctor at my appointment. But I wasn't sure I could get the question out without crying, so I held off. I was determined to appear strong and in control at each of these appointments. I didn't realize my doctors were waiting for me to ask. I was haunted by the numbers I used to type in papers for Gene when he was in surgery residency. Back before personal computers, I would help Gene by typing up his research papers on breast cancer. I clearly remember the survival rate for some breast cancer was 50 percent. This terrified me.

A couple weeks and many doctor's appointments went by before I finally asked Gene the question. We were driving home from yet another appointment. It felt like talk of breast cancer dominated our lives. We had the biopsy results and treatment plan outlined and had met with all my specialists. We were ready for surgery, and I finally asked him what my chance of survival was. I held my breath and prayed that I wouldn't cry and make him feel bad.

He said that if the lymph nodes were not involved and nothing changed in the pathology report after surgery, my chance of survival at five years was 85 percent. I exhaled. That didn't sound so bad. Then he went on to explain that if I completed chemo, radiation, and Herceptin infusions (phase three) and took tamoxifen, my survival rate increased a bit. Woo-hoo! That is like going from a B to an A. When I asked about the numbers I typed in reports nearly thirty years ago, Gene explained all the advances in treatment and targeted chemotherapy and how survival rates have increased dramatically since his residency days.

I asked Gene why doctors don't tell you your chance of survival from the start. He explained that there are so many variables and each specialist looks at survival rates differently. And then he made a very good point. He told me that if a patient is in the 15 percent that doesn't have a good outcome, they feel cheated by the numbers, and the 85 percent survival rate means nothing to them. Point taken. So I was careful to keep this in perspective.

At my postop appointment, my surgeon encouraged me to talk to my oncologist about this when I was ready. I put it on the back burner because I felt I had enough information to start treatment, but as I prepared to write this post, I decided to ask her. Gene was with me at the appointment, so I knew I would have a second set of ears to process the information. I was surprised to find my hands shaking as I asked the question.

Here is where we get to see the difference in philosophies among specialties. When I asked my oncologist what my survival rate was, she clarified and said, "You want to know what your chance of cure is." Okay, I'm good with that. She told me they had a computer model they could plug all my specific information into (size and type of tumor, hormone receptive and HER2/neu positive, stage, etc.), and it would give me a chart. I love charts! I got all excited knowing that I would have a piece of paper to look at.

After processing the information on the chart that my doctor gave me for a few days and talking with Gene, I have decided this is a decision matrix rather than a survival chart. It outlines what the survival and relapse numbers are if you (1) only have surgery, (2) have surgery and only hormone therapy, (3) have surgery and only chemo, and finally (4) have all three: surgery, chemo, and hormone therapy. What the model does not show is increased cure due to radiation and Herceptin infusions. Are you confused yet? For the numbers people, here is what the bottom line says (again, this is for my specific diagnosis):

- Seventy-nine out of one hundred women (with my diagnosis) are alive and without cancer in ten years.
- Seventeen out of one hundred women relapse within ten years.
- Four out of one hundred women die of other causes within ten years.

As I look at the printout, I think this is a great tool for deciding whether to do chemo, hormone therapy, or both. You then need to have a conversation with your radiologist on what the benefit of radiation is for your particular diagnosis. This conversation is a blast and filled with even more numbers. In the end, I don't think there is a good, solid number for my survival rate. But if attitude has anything to do with it, I have this thing licked!

That Was Easy

Someone made a comment to me the other day that had me wondering if I have made a mistake by sharing my amusing stories of surviving cancer. Their comment was, "I can't believe how easily you got through your treatment for cancer." The comment threw me, and I had to think about my reply. I would never disrespect or dishonor those who have gone through breast cancer by implying that it was easy for me. On the contrary, this is the toughest thing I have had to do in my life. And it has been a very long fight.

Through diagnosis and treatment, I fought tears, fear, uncertainty, anger, fatigue, side effects, nausea, and all the other emotions that cancer patients face, but one thing was important to me—I wanted to make my battle as easy as possible for my family and friends. And let's face it: my sense of humor was bound to come out like it always does. I have been turning disasters into funny stories to entertain my friends for most of my life. That is why my husband jokingly refers to me as Pollyanna.

When I first learned of my fifteen-month treatment plan, I was afraid that I would be nauseated and fatigued for the entire time. I don't function well when I'm nauseated, so this was a huge concern for me. But I have to admit, my next thought was, "Well, maybe I will lose some weight!" So throughout my treatment, if I was upright (standing) and not nauseated, when someone asked how my day was going, I would reply, "I'm fantastic!" I would watch huge grins come over that person's face as this bald woman with a sparkle in her eye proclaimed she was fantastic.

I remember one grocery store clerk saying, "I'm going to remember that. You inspire me."

Only a small number of people got to see me on the bad days when the sofa became my best friend. This close circle of family and friends watched over me while I rested, and they took on the cooking, the cleaning, and my work. Sometimes I felt like I was just trying to live from one chemo appointment to another. On my good days, which were many, I would hold Gene's hand at the end of the day and say, "I had a good day today," and he would smile and say, "I'm glad."

Every cancer patient is entitled to choose how to go through treatment. Some may feel they need to hide from the world. Some may surround themselves with friends. Some may cry or feel that life is unfair. I understand and respect all of those feelings. But for a lucky few of us, we see the humor in the world and choose to not put our lives on hold. We shake and rattle the bars and laugh when our friends join us in celebrating each day God gave us.

So no. It wasn't easy. But it sure was funny a lot of the time!

The Mentors

One of the perks of being diagnosed with breast cancer is that nearly every community has a breast cancer survivors group. These groups meet regularly and share feelings and stories about their experiences with surviving cancer. Shortly after I started letting people know I had been diagnosed with cancer, I was contacted by the local survivors group and invited to join their meetings. Their meetings are held monthly on a Tuesday night in a community about twenty miles from my house.

Since I was really feeling the effects of my chemo treatments, Gene drove me to the meeting and encouraged me to stay as long as I wanted. I think I lasted an hour before the combination of fatigue and nausea had me making my excuses, and I called Gene to come pick me up. He must have been worried about me, because he was only a few blocks away. So the combination of distance and side effects made the survivors group unworkable at that stage of my journey.

After thinking about it for a while, I decided I wanted online support. I communicate online daily, and I felt this would meet my needs better than having to travel to town. I just needed a couple of people I could talk to who would be just an e-mail away. I talked with some friends, and I was connected to two amazing women who I had never met.

My first mentor was Julie. Julie lives about two-and-a-half hours away from me and is the sister of my friend Joanne. Julie was diagnosed with cancer about ten years ago, while she was in her forties. She has a great sense of humor and would answer the most personal questions even when I was too nervous or embarrassed to ask them. This is one of the great benefits of having cyber mentors. I could talk about things that I might have hesitated to talk about in person. Julie's e-mail responses were full of laughs and insight. She even sent me a photo of herself in pink pajamas drinking a glass of wine for me. She was the first person to tell me about chemo brain and the advantage I would have in using it as an excuse the rest of my life. Other people might become forgetful as they age, but we could claim chemo brain.

My second mentor was Chris. She lives about forty-five minutes from me and is the mother of one of my son's friends. The odd coincidence is that when Chris was diagnosed with breast cancer about five years ago, I made a meal for her and sent it over to her house with my son. I had never met Chris but, knowing that her children were similar ages to my children, felt such empathy for her. Chris, too, had a great sense of humor and encouraged me with stories of using cancer to get out of things while I could. She also gave me practical advice about the cumulative effects of chemo and told me what to expect.

Both Julie and Chris told me they were honored when I asked them to be my breast cancer mentors. But in fact, I am the one who was honored to have them as mentors. These ladies stuck with me for two years of treatment and reconstruction. I had the privilege of meeting them after I finished phase two of chemo, and they will be my friends for life.

Mr. Potato Head

We took a family trip last weekend to celebrate the end of reconstruction. When we got to the airport, Danielle, leaned over and whispered to me, "I don't mean to embarrass you, but did you bring your tooth?" I tried not to laugh as I assured her that I had packed my tooth *and* my hearing aids *and* my new glasses. It is getting harder to travel as I have to remember to pack all my its and bits. I sort of feel like Mr. Potato Head with all the interchangeable parts. How embarrassing it could be to travel with a piece missing!

My "tooth" is a temporary tooth embedded on a retainer that serves no function other than to keep me from getting double takes when I smile. The dry mouth caused by chemo accelerated some decay and caused me to lose two teeth. Naturally, one of those teeth had to be a front tooth. When the dentist pulled it, I grinned at him and asked, "Does this affect my smile?" The dental assistant cracked up and then apologized for laughing. I didn't mind her laughter. It was funny. If I'm really good (or lucky), I will get my permanent tooth by Christmas.

The hearing aids were a significant financial investment from a few years ago that rarely saw the light of day and I mostly kept in my closet. I wore them only when I wanted to hear what other people had to say. As it turns out, that isn't very often. Unfortunately, near the end of treatment, I noticed that my hearing had gotten worse, and I was missing more conversations than I was catching. My mistakes in ordering things at restaurants that I didn't know I was ordering have become family folklore. My trick of nodding or saying okay when I don't hear someone has resulted in some very amusing moments. The kids laugh and Gene just shakes his head when I shrug and pretend it wasn't my fault. I got the hearing levels turned up on my hearing aids and now try to wear them when I leave the house. The best part of hearing aids is that when I get tired of listening to people, I just take the batteries out and claim that they are dead.

And my eyesight changes have resulted in new glasses and sunglasses. But I was tired of the old ones anyway. The past two months have been a series of appointments to get all my new its and bits so I'm once again complete. Now all I have to do is remember to take everything with me when I leave the house—but I'm not taking spare batteries for the hearing aids!

Serial Numbers

I had an appointment with my dentist today to take the final impressions for my dental implant. As the dentist checked everything out and the hygienist prepared the gooey substance to form the impression, I asked the dentist if my implant had a number engraved on it. He took my questions seriously and, after inserting the tray of paste in my mouth, began to explain that implants do have numbers but they aren't engraved on the actual implant. After a long explanation and three minutes of waiting for the paste to harden, he removed the tray and asked if he had answered my question. I told him I was just curious since I had a collection of signed and numbered parts and wondered if I was going to have to keep track of this number as well.

We then entertained ourselves discussing whether manufacturers ever recall implants like they do cars. I can just see myself watching that story on the news, then logging into a website to see if my implant has been recalled. How long and where do people actually keep these implant numbers? The nurse handed me a card after my reconstruction surgeries with my breast implant numbers on it, but I haven't determined what to name the file where I keep it. And I kid you not, the implant card instructs me to register my implant online. Are they kidding? Isn't this some sort of breach of patient privacy? Do I really want to get on a website and register my boobs?

Our discussion turned back to finishing my dental implant, and the dentist told me it would take about two-and-a-half weeks to get my final crown. I told him that I had been really good this year and had asked Santa if I could have my front tooth for Christmas. The dentist told me that I must not have been that good, because my tooth wouldn't be ready until December 30. Bummer. Rather than focusing on my disappointment, I think I will spend my energy on coming up with a creative file name for my implant numbers. Maybe "Its and Bits"…

Limited Potential

Several weeks after my final surgery, our new pet, Miss Luci, was needing some playtime. She was holding me to the pet adoption contract that said I would make sure she got regular exercise, despite my doctor's note that said I was still recovering. Luci had been as patient as she could be after my surgery, given her attention span, but on this sunny day, she was insistent that we go outside and play. As I considered my options, I quickly ruled out her favorite game of tug-of-war as I was sure that she would either pull my arm out of the socket or rip some sutures. Luci is an eight-year-old German shepherd who thinks she is three years old. When she plays tug-of-war, she wins.

So I settled on her second-favorite toy, which is a squeaky tennis ball, and headed out to the yard with her bouncing up and down at my side. Luci's eyes sparkled. We reached the driveway, and I pulled back my arm to throw the ball. I took a deep breath and heaved the ball as hard as I could…and it landed at my feet. Poor Luci. Her look of disappointment was something to see. She looked up at me with those deep-brown eyes like, "Really?" My face, on the other hand, showed confusion. How could my arm have failed me?

It was about this time that I remembered my first meeting with the plastic surgeon as he discussed my potential surgery. During this meeting, the surgeon explained that if I proceeded with this surgery, there would be some things I would no longer be able to do. He mentioned that I could no longer be an Olympic-class rower. I sighed at the time and mumbled, "Another dream crushed," which made Gene snicker. I do remember thinking that I should be paying more attention, but my mind wandered to friends inviting me to join a rowing exercise class and my response: "I'm sorry. My doctor has advised me not to row." Or what if I'm shipwrecked and have to evacuate to the lifeboats and it is my turn to row? Would a doctor's note get me out of it? Oh, the possibilities.

Now that I have completed all the surgeries and recovery, I'm finding that I have limited potential. There are times when my body fails me, and that surprises me. For example, I will never be able to play Frisbee golf. When I throw a Frisbee with my right hand, it is likely to go anywhere. I have had the Frisbee end up in a tree, behind me, at my feet, and on the roof. Miss Luci looks ever hopeful when I pick up her Frisbee, but now she won't even return it to me. I remember the day both of us stood looking up in the tree with perplexed expressions on our faces. I now see her look of disdain as she carries it with her for the entire walk. She would rather carry it herself than give it to me to get stuck in a tree.

I have also had to set aside any dream of being a swimsuit model. I have a patchwork of scars on my chest and back that would be difficult to Photoshop out. I thought about applying for disability, but I'm sure the first question would be, "Were you *ever* a swimsuit model?" I doubt I could fake my way through that interview.

And finally, I can no longer be a backseat driver...or a spy. It is impossible. When I try to look over my shoulder, I get back spasms that make me whimper. Spies can't whimper. I read that somewhere. So whoever is driving me is just going to have to go it alone, without my help. And the CIA is going to have to recruit someone else. While I may have limited potential, I do have an unlimited sense of humor and imagination. I think I will be fine.

Journey's End

Now that my treatment and reconstruction surgeries are over, my journey with breast cancer has come to an end. I have enjoyed sharing my stories with you, but now it is time for me to set my focus forward. As I look to the future, I know I am stronger than when I started this journey, and I know that laughter helped me not only survive but win my battle with cancer. Thank you for walking with me and encouraging me along the way.

ABOUT THE AUTHOR

Kathy started writing in high school and hoped to become a journalist, until she discovered that sticking to the facts was boring. She also majored in accounting for only one semester for the same reason. After retiring from the phone company at the age of twenty-six, Kathy spent the majority of her life as a compulsive volunteer helping nonprofit organizations with membership and financial campaigns. She opened a website design and promotion business using the skills she developed while volunteering. But she always returned to writing.

Though she considers herself a Texan at heart, she now lives in Iowa with her husband, Gene, and walking companion, Luci Dog. Her three grown children are "off the family payroll" and successful in their communities. If she's not working on her latest blog, you can find her reading, creating websites, traveling, or laughing with her friends.

Made in the USA
San Bernardino, CA
29 February 2016